SUCCESSFUL FASTING

Rid your body of unwanted toxins, revitalize your internal organs and restore the natural biological balance that is essential to healthy living.

About the author

Dr Hellmut Lützner MD worked at the world-famous Buchinger Fasting Clinic for twelve years. Since 1975, he has been the chief medical officer of the Kurpark Fasting Clinic in Überlingen on Lake Constance on the German/Swiss border.

SUCCESSFUL FASTING

The easy way to cleanse your body of its poisons

Dr Hellmut Lützner
Translated from the German by Ann E. Woollcombe

THORSONS PUBLISHING GROUP

This third edition, newly translated from *Wie neugeboren durch Fasten* (1988 edition), published 1990

First published in the UK as *The Secrets of Successful Fasting* 1978
Second revised edition 1984

Original German edition published by Gräfe und Unzer GmbH, Munich 1988

British Library Cataloguing in Publication Data

Lutzner, Hellmut
  Successful fasting.
  1. Fasting
  I. Title
  613.2'5

  ISBN 0-7225-2130-8

Published by Thorsons Publishers Limited,
Wellingborough, Northamptonshire NN8 2RQ, England

Typeset by Harper Phototypesetters Limited, Northampton, England
Printed in Great Britain by The Bath Press, Bath, Avon

10 9 8 7 6 5 4 3 2

Contents

Chapter 6: Clinical therapeutic fasting 72

Introduction

This book tells you what fasting is all about: the most effective and at the same time the safest way to lose weight, the most effective and the safest way to cleanse your body of poisons it may have been accumulating for years. Beautiful skin and elastic tissues are welcome side-effects.

This is the proven medical guide for healthy people who wish to experience a week's fast on their own - be it at home or during a holiday. This guide gives you exact instructions about preparing the fast, how to live during the fasting period, how to break the fast and how to resume normal eating patterns step by step. It will help you to live your fasting experience safely, without hunger pangs and in full physical fitness.

Chapter 1
What is fasting?

Eating and not eating are like waking and sleeping, like tension and relaxation: two opposite poles between which most human life is lived.

Eating by day and fasting by night are so much part of life's rhythm that no one gives the matter a second thought. Only if we eat late at night do we realize in the morning that we are not hungry. Our body gives us the signal that the fasting period is not yet over, that it has been extended.

There is a good reason why the first meal of the day is called 'breakfast'. It is the meal that 'breaks the fast'. If we do not fast during the night, there is no real reason to 'break the fast' in the morning.

People need about twelve to fourteen hours a day to be awake, to work, to eat, to be in contact with their environment, to act and react. Therefore they have ten to twelve hours left during the night for their metabolism, i.e. the processing of bodily substances. The energy needed for this process is supplied from the body's own energy deposits. During the fasting period at night, the body takes care of itself. We sleep and keep still. Rest, comfort and warmth help us to live off our own resources. These three things are the decisive requirements for all fasting; we will come back to them again and again in this book.

Fasting and illness

Just as when we are sleeping, we need rest, comfort and warmth when we are ill. We also need solitude. A feverish child refuses to eat and asks only for cold drinks; a sick dog will hide in its kennel and not eat for days. Instinctively, sick creatures do the right thing: they fast.

The sick organism needs time to itself in order to get well. The energy necessary to rebuild its sick cells and to generate new ones is supplied from its own nutritional resources. By fasting, the body saves the energy required by digestion, which represents 30 per cent of the total energy expended. The energy thus made available is used in the healing process.

This instinctive fasting during a fever or any other illness is nature's wonderful self-help method. We know for certain that both fever and fasting are highly effective in healing illness in an otherwise healthy person. They:

- *destroy bacteria;*
- *stop the spreading and growth of viruses;*
- *increase the immunity of the blood and of the cells;*
- *intensify the elimination of toxins.*

Fasting and physical fitness

Perhaps you know from experience that strength, speed, perseverance and concentration are by no means a function of your food intake. On the contrary, you think better and more quickly when your stomach is not full.

What mountain climber would eat just before his climb? If he leaves at three o'clock in the morning, he will climb for three, four or even five hours during the night's extended fasting period. Only then will he eat breakfast. A runner will never reach her peak performance if she eats just before the start of the race.

These examples demonstrate that a person does not normally live from 'hand to mouth', that we do not get our strength directly from eating. We get our energy from the nutritional reserves stored in our own bodies. They can be tapped immediately, contrary to the energy available from food which needs time and energy to be digested.

Ask yourself the following questions:

- *When am I particularly energetic?*
- *When did I last eat before that?*
- *Did I eat a lot? A little? Nothing at all?*
- *Did I need stimulants such as coffee, tea, Coca-Cola, nicotine, alcohol?*
- *When am I at my best physically?*

There is a further point which helps us prove that energy is not directly derived from food: not only during, but even *after* physical exertion we do not feel the need for food. First of all we quench our thirst, and only then do we feel hungry.

Sportsmen are aware of the relationship between fitness and fasting; they know they can perform by drawing on the energy stored in the nutritional reserves of their own bodies. We repeat: the metabolism during fasting avoids loss of energy through digestion and makes this saved energy available to ensure a maximum performance.

It is even possible to go without food for days, indeed weeks, and still accomplish great feats. The Swedish physician Otto Karl Aly reports of a fasting march undertaken by 20 Swedes who were convinced that not only is it possible to live off one's own nutritional reserves, but one is also capable of strenuous exercise during fasting time. The men walked from Göteborg to Stockholm, covering 500 kilometres in 10 days, i.e. 50 kilometres a day. They lived on a little fruit juice and about 3 litres of water per day. Dr Aly reports, that despite an average weight loss of 5 to 7 kilograms, the men were in great shape and in high spirits. Nor were they exhausted, but arrived in Stockholm with increased energy and perseverance.

Fasting and feasting

What would life be without parties? Eating is an important element of all celebrations. All over the world, feasts do not just satisfy our hunger; indeed they are characterized by gluttony, exaggeration and are always a luxury. They are not a response to the need for food, but rather for social contacts and enjoyment, for sensual pleasures and the appetite for the unusual. Feasts become games played with knives and forks and wine glasses.

Whatever the next day may bring, be it a hangover, upset stomach or simply a lack of appetite – why not fast on that day? The body needs a sensible compensation. Why not listen to it?

It would be good sense not to eat after the feast until you really feel hungry again, be it after some hours or even days.

Fasting = life without food

The changeover from eating to fasting happens by itself. The programmes run automatically. The proper *changeover from energy programme I to energy programme II* is prepared for by:

● *the knowledge that humans are able to fast*

● *confidence in the safety of this natural measure*
● *the voluntary decision to fast.*

The changeover is initiated by a thorough cleansing of the bowels. It is the signal for the changeover and the beginning of the fast.

The real acceptance of the fast occurs during the first fasting days, when first-time fasters make the amazing discovery that *they are not hungry, feel well and are functioning as usual.* This discovery results in growing confidence in the body's ability to look after itself. The experience that life without food is possible gives fasters the inner security non-fasters always admire.

The two energy programmes

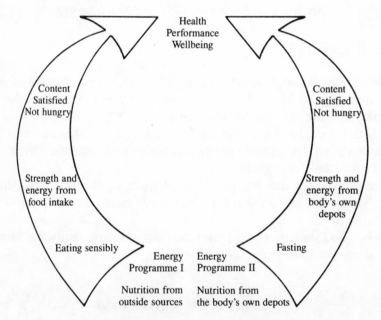

Living with the body's two energy programmes

Hunger is the body's way of signalling: 'I am expecting food. I am prepared to take in food. I am producing saliva and stomach juices. My metabolism is switched to Energy Programme I.' If food as energy source is not forthcoming, the body's expectations are deceived. The hunger signal turns to the disagreeable, indeed,

14

torturing experience we call 'hunger.' It is a feeling in the pit of the stomach which continues and grows until we cannot think of anything else. If it becomes serious, the metabolism may react with dizziness, nausea and weakness, sometimes even with shaking and perspiration. Even a glass of juice can remedy the situation in five to ten minutes. Solid food has a more lasting effect.

It should be noted that appetite or hunger are not necessarily a desire for food. They may express a longing for love, for comfort, for recognition by others and a better self-image.

Countless people become obese or their metabolism goes wrong, because they subconsciously try to compensate their emotional needs by eating, drinking or smoking.

It is now easy to understand why fasters do not feel hungry. They have changed over to Energy Programme II. They do not feel hungry because their inner energy sources keep them well supplied. As long as the inner nutritional stores are not exhausted, they can fast. In a healthy person, all organs continue to function as always.

You may now understand why it is so difficult to skip a meal or eat less than usual, for example on a 1000-calorie diet. The body is switched to Energy Programme I, and does not get sufficient food, so it starves.

Life on Energy Programme II, which means not eating at all, is actually a great deal easier.

Everyone has the ability to change over to fasting, but this ability has to be practised. A body that is used to fasting can change over much faster when there is no food intake than a body unused to fasting. To forego a meal does not present a problem to experienced fasters. They even manage to change over to a half-way position between Energy Programme I and Energy Programme II, in other words to live on a reduced diet and cover their energy needs partly from food and partly from the body's inner depots without feeling hungry. This happens already during the post-fasting period after a short fasting week. The rule of thumb is:

Fasting is not starving. Anyone who starves is not fasting.

It should now have become clear that 'fasting = life without food' is a natural part of life. It seems strange indeed that many people do not realize this. The idea of living without eating, and even working during that time, seems inconceivable to them.

They are afraid of illness, indeed even death. Such prejudices die hard. Yet we only have to observe nature in order to know better.

Fasting in the animal world

Fasting for weeks or even months is a normal part of the life rhythm of many animals that live in the wild. It is the ability to survive that is planned by nature. In autumn, mountain animals such as ibex, chamois, deer and marmots acquire a heavy layer of fat which allows them to survive a long time. While the marmot goes into hibernation and does not expend much energy, the ibex and the chamois as well as the deer must fight against snow and ice and the cold. The fact that this fasting period is also their mating period, with the males' fierce battles against their rivals and the females' period of fertility, should convince even the sceptics that fasting does not mean diminished vitality, quite the contrary.

There is a similarity in the lives of birds and fish. The salmon does not take food during its long journey upstream, nor during the subsequent spawning time. Migratory birds eat more than they need during the second half of summer. They often have twice their normal weight when they fly south. Thanks to their energy, stored as fat, they are able to fly up to 500 kilometres non-stop. After this top performance, their weight is back to normal.

Wolves are known to live without food for days and months and still cover long stretches. Almost all predatory animals eat when they find food; when they don't manage to find their prey, they live on the nutritional reserves stored in their own bodies.

Origins of human fasting

In the same way as animals, humans in the distant past depended on their innate ability to survive on stored nutrients. It was a biological necessity for survival. Without this ability, whole peoples would have disappeared.

Survival is still possible if the lack of food exists over a long period of time, even if important substances have been exhausted. It takes a long time to die of starvation.

Indigenous peoples in Africa and Australia still have to adapt to their sparse environment just as they did thousands of years ago. Times during which they can eat their fill and store food in their bodies give way to times where there is no food at all.

The history of the Hunza is a good example of the fact that fasting can mean more than the possibility of survival. This small group of about 10000 people lives in the high valleys of the central Himalayan mountains. Until a few decades ago, the Hunza were completely cut off from the outside world. In his book, *The Hunza*, Dr Ralph Bircher tells an amazing tale. The fields of the high valleys did not yield enough food to supply the people the whole year round, so until they could harvest the barley in March, the whole population fasted for weeks, sometimes for as long as two months. The Hunza remained content and cheerful. They accomplished most of the work for the whole year. They tended their fields and repaired the drainage ditches which had been destroyed by avalanches. The Hunza knew no medical doctors and had no need for policemen; their lives were lived according to the laws of nature.

Nowadays, the valley has become accessible. The Hunza men serve as soldiers in India, or they work there. Staples such as sugar, flour and tinned foods are imported; the people are no longer 'starving'. The country of the Hunza now suffers from the typical illnesses of civilization: tooth decay, appendicitis, gall bladder trouble, obesity, colds, diabetes, to name just a few. Not only do the people need doctors, they also need policemen. The health of their bodies as well as of their behaviour and their thinking has been destroyed.

This example may allow us to understand the origins of religious fasts. People give thanks for the God-given ability to survive and for not starving. The fast is experienced as a way to gain inner peace, to find one's way to maturity. The great religious founders Moses, Christ, Buddha and Mohammed found the basic key to existence during long, voluntary fasts.

Is there anyone today, continuously surrounded by food, who can understand the deeper meaning of such a solitary fast, a voluntary reununciation of food? As soon as we are forced to fast, we react with hunger and rebellion. Even the Christian church has not been successful in its fasting rules: prescribed fast days or rules for Lent were circumvented or ignored, leading to more and more dispensations on the part of the Church, often based on fear of injuring one's health. What is left are meaningless canons.

We should strive for an unprejudiced rediscovery of fasting. The best way to do so is to experience the fast yourself. It is a personal experience that is available to everyone.

The prerequisites for a successful fast are openness to new experiences, readiness to try fasting and the perseverance to stick to it.

Fasting is:

- *a natural form of living*
- *life based on the body's own nutrients*
- *the body's ability to function normally based on its inner resources*
- *a way of life for independent people able to make their own decisions*
- *something that affects the whole person, each single cell, soul and spirit*
- *the best opportunity to stay physically fit or to get back in shape. Furthermore, it helps us to change our way of life if this is necessary.*

The five basic rules of fasting

Rule 1. Do not eat for one or two or more weeks. Only drink tea, vegetable broth, fruit or vegetable juices and water, more than you need to quench your thirst.

Rule 2. Leave out everything not necessary to living. That means all things that have become enjoyable habits, but would harm the body during fasting: nicotine and alcohol in every form, sweets and coffee; medication unless essential. Diuretics, appetite depressants and laxatives should never be taken.

Rule 3. Free yourself as far as possible from your everyday routine. Get out of professional and family obligations. Stay away from the telephone and your appointment book. Renounce the newspapers, radio and television. Instead of outside stimuli listen to yourself. Follow directives that come from within yourself.

Rule 4. Behave naturally: listen to your body and its needs. If you are tired, get some sleep. If you need exercise, walk, swim, do sports. Do all the things you like - read, dance, listen to music, enjoy your hobbies.

Rule 5. Keep strict toilet habits. Empty the bowels regularly, flush the kidneys, perspire, breathe properly, take care of your skin and mucous membranes.

Fasting is not:

- *starving*
- *deprivation or want*
- *eating less*
- *forgoing meat on Fridays: that would only be abstinence*
- *the fanaticism of some sect*
- *necessarily tied to religious practices.*

Ways to fast

Water fasting – Drinking only good spring or mineral water, 1½ litres per day for people whose weight is normal, 2-3 litres for people who are overweight.

Zero diet – is a fast restricted to water during which vitamin and mineral tablets are taken. It is usually only undertaken in a hospital.

Tea fasting – three times daily, 2 cups of various herbal teas (unsweetened). Water is taken intermittently. Tea fasting also has zero calories, but it has an advantage over water fasting in that warm drinks are consumed with the added benefit of the herbs.

Gruel fasting – especially suited to people with delicate stomachs or bowels.

Fresh juice fasting – 3 to 5 times daily, one glass of freshly squeezed fruit or vegetable juice. Water is taken intermittently.

Whey fast – one litre of whey spread over one day, supplemented with herbal teas and fresh juices.

Buchinger method – with tea, juice and hot vegetable broths. This fast has proved highly effective and has been used for decades in the renowned Buchinger clinics. We recommend it as the most suitable form of fasting at home.

Fasting on one's own

Take advantage of the many opportunities which will arise almost every day.

Do not force yourself to eat if you are not hungry. Many people have no appetite in the morning. Therefore their first meal should be at noon (morning fast). Fast after

What we can gain through fasting

- *Fasting is the quickest, easiest and safest method of losing extra weight.*
- *Through fasting we can learn to enjoy eating moderately and to avoid the excesses of overconsumption, so typical of our era.*
- *Fasting helps fight dependency on alcohol or drugs.*
- *Through fasting, the tissues become decongested and purified of toxic substances making them supple and no longer painful.*
- *Fasting tones all connective tissue and gives you a clearer skin.*
- *Fasting is one of the few successful biological measures for detoxification in our polluted environment.*
- *Fasting maintains physical and mental fitness, especially during menopause for women and for men around forty.*
- *Fasting cannot stop the ageing process, but it helps to prevent premature ageing.*
- *Fasting as an early therapeutic measure is constantly gaining in importance as laboratory techniques are now able to identify symptoms of serious diseases at an early stage.*
- *Therapeutic fasting in a clinic is the most effective and safest way to treat diet-related diseases of the metabolism. Dr Buchinger called it the 'royal road to health' in many chronic or acute diseases. Every physician who has fasting experience will support this theory.*

you have overindulged, after celebrations, when you have an upset stomach or diarrhoea. Fast until you feel hungry again. Fast when you have a fever, flu, tonsillitis or bronchitis accompanied by fever.

Plan a short fast of five days the next time you have a free or relatively easy week.

Do not confuse this fasting week (5 days' fast + three days returning to normal eating) with therapeutic fasting! Therapeutic fasting requires the conditions outlined in the section on fasting in a clinic. The 5-day fast is the quickest way in which to become familiar with the phenomenon of fasting and to get some idea of what results are possible through a therapeutic fast of two to four weeks. It is best to start off easily and thus be encouraged to fast for a longer period later on. To begin your first fast of a few days you need only a little courage and interest in learning something new.

Chapter 2
A week-long fast for healthy people

Fasting at home – who can safely do it?

This fast may be carried out by all physically fit people who know that they are in good health and are willing to exercise self-discipline. Older people, young people 14 years of age and older, and people who are handicapped may fast, if their bodies function normally. Healthy pregnant or breastfeeding women can in theory fast as well, but this may not be advisable in today's polluted environment. As long as we cannot be sure that the detoxifying process will not harm the baby, it would be better to fast *after* the baby is weaned or before becoming pregnant.

When is it best not to fast at home?

- *If you still have doubts about fasting after reading this book.*
- *If you suffer from long-term depression or are psychologically unstable.*
- *If you are still weak after an illness or operation. If you are exhausted, nervous and agitated you should wait until you feel better.*
- *If you are on medication. It would be better for you to fast in a hospital or clinic.*
- *If you are not sure you are healthy. Consult your family doctor and discuss the risk factors.*
- *If you do not consider yourself in good health, for example, due to high or low blood pressure or to a chronic ailment, you should not fast without the advice of a physician. Read carefully the section on therapeutic fasting.*

The best way to fast

The easiest way to fast is with a group of like-minded people. If you are within a group of friends, fasting can be a very exciting experience. However, all fasters should have their own refuge where they can at times be alone. The group can meet regularly, exchange experiences and share some common activities. In a group of fasters, you benefit from multiple experience, your interpersonal relationships are strengthened and the mutual support helps you to succeed. Before you start your 5-day fast, you might like to consult with a physician who has fasting experience and is willing to guide the group.

The same rules that apply to a group of fasters apply on a smaller scale to fasting with a partner. The experience of fasting together; coming to terms with yourself and your partner, and helping one another, can strengthen the relationship between two people. But the same rule applies: both partners should have the opportunity to be alone sometimes, both physically and mentally.

Fasting alone is much harder. It requires a great deal of self-discipline, courage and the ability to come to terms with yourself. If you make it through a 5-day fast on your own, you can justifiably be proud of yourself.

Where and when?

You can fast wherever you are comfortable, wherever you feel warm and sheltered. This may be in your own home, a holiday apartment, at the home of good friends, in a hut in the mountains, on a boat or in your garden.

Wherever you feel at home, where you can pursue your favourite sport or be lazy if that is what you want, in short, in the surroundings you like best.

You should fast where you have peace and quiet and where you are left alone. No rushing about, no deadlines to meet! Fasters often feel the need to crawl into their shell.

Fasting at home

If you plan to fast at home, you have to be aware that here all your old habits of eating and drinking lie in wait for you. They are in all the things and in the people around you. As is the case for all of us, there are thousands of invisible threads tying you to your usual environment, to kitchen, cellar, refrigerator, dining room table and liquor cabinet. However, what will interfere most with fasting at home – and you must be aware of this – are the know-it-alls: prejudiced neighbours and relatives, who will give you lots of unsolicited advice. You will hear from all sides 'but only the other day I read in the paper . . .', 'taste a bit of this . . . surely it can't do you any harm!' or 'you're bound to make yourself ill if you go on like this!' And all this while you, the poor faster, are desperately trying to find peace and quiet.

However well-intended, this kind of advice is much more disturbing to the faster than the sight of someone cooking in the kitchen, for example, or the children coming home hungry from school.

To sum up, fasting at home is not necessarily the ideal situation, but you must choose for yourself which is the most comfortable, warm and sheltered place. If your own home meets these criteria, then you should fast at home and you will be successful.

Fasting on holiday

Include your eight days of fasting early on in your holiday plans. It would be ideal if you could take a week off. If that is not possible, you should at least try to plan your fast at a time where you are not overtaxed in your work and when you can avoid social obligations.

Fasting and being free of obligations really ought to go together. That means being free of all the demands of the exhausting daily grind, free of stress, noise and pollution.

Treat yourself to a fasting holiday! Experienced fasters know that fasting is best then. For your nervous system, it means switching from the daily battle to relaxation. This is an important prerequisite for proper fasting and the best guarantee of success.

Fasting while you work

It is also possible to fast during everyday life. I know many people who do this routinely. They tell me that the activities of everyday life divert one's thoughts from eating and drinking. However, fasting during a working day requires greater discipline and self-assurance. Those who are already familiar with fasting know what they can expect of themselves. For the first-time faster, holidays are undoubtedly easier.

Apart from the many temptations to which you will be exposed, and the attitude of your colleagues trying to break your determination, there are other dangers I should point out:

- *You slow down during a fast: everything takes longer to do.*
- *The blood circulation is not as stable as usual. In most cases, this is only for a few hours. But what if those are the most important hours?*
- *Fasters are usually more sensitive and thus more vulnerable to personal insults and less able to stand up to injustices.*
- *If you drive a car you should know that your reactions may be slower and your ability to concentrate reduced.*

On no account should you fast while working if you have a job that places heavy demands on you or if you are responsible for the welfare of others, or if you have to handle equipment, for example a lathe, or a crane, or drive a taxi or a bus.

Where to go for advice

If you feel you are not in completely good health, you should consult your doctor before starting a fast. You cannot expect him or her to have fasting experience, but you can expect to get a report on your general health as well as advice on the reaction to medication while on a fast. During the actual fasting week, any physician who has experience with fasting will be glad to be of help. Before contacting the doctor, however, you might check to see if your question is not already answered in this book. Consult the index.

Anyone who has had fasting experience can be a great support to the healthy faster who embarks on this venture for the first time. An exchange of experiences is all-important, and you have the reassuring feeling that there is someone who knows what it is all about and who can advise you if need be.

Preparing for the fast

Shopping

For the first six days (5 fast days + the day before) you will need:

- *Three pounds of fruit for the 'fruit day' or fresh vegetables for the 'raw vegetable day' or 150g (5½ oz) brown rice for your 'rice day'.*
- *½ pound of linseed, shredded, often available as Linusit in your health food store.*
- *5-10 bottles of still mineral water – not necessary if you have good spring or tap water.*

- *15 sachets of herbal tea, various kinds. Loose tea is better or fresh leaves from your garden; mild black tea or Ginseng tea, if you tend to have low blood pressure.*
- *1½ litres (2½ pints) of fruit juice (your favourite kind, in any combination).*
- *Vegetables and herbs for the vegetable broths (see page 29).*
- *2 large bottles of vegetable juice (1½ litres/2½ pints) from your health food store or 5 small ones, a different one for each day.*
- *1 bottle of sauerkraut juice. It's best to ask for advice at your health food store and choose high quality juices that contain plenty of vitamins but little sugar.*
- *5 lemons.*
- *40g Glaubersalts (sodium sulphate) weighed precisely by your pharmacy.*
- *50g Epsom salts (magnesium sulphate).*
- *An enema bag, hose and rectal tube (should be in every medicine cabinet).*

It is best to put off the shopping for your post-fasting diet until the last day of your fast. It is fun to shop while you are still fasting, and it will increase your anticipation of eating again.

Starting with a clean slate

Take care of all burdensome tasks and outstanding obligations. Eat and drink normally. Don't stuff yourself. There is no reason for it. Or perhaps you are afraid? Give away any food you have on hand, or lock it up and give the key to the neighbours.

Getting ready

- *clothing a little warmer than usual*
- *enough underwear for more frequent changes*
- *track suit*
- *hot water bottle*
- *enema bag, rectal tube or rubber syringe*
- *skin oil*
- *brush for dry brushing*
- *linen towel.*

Chapter 3
The fasting week

The day before

Eat little! Eat plenty of fresh, uncooked vegetables or fruit. Three times a day, take one tablespoon of linseed mixed with yoghurt or apple purée. These substances will become gelatinous and absorb the toxins and waste in the intestines. The following are three samples of strict diets which will be useful to overweight people wanting to lose two or three pounds quickly at any given time, or for people who want to reduce their blood pressure or give their heart a rest.

Fruit day
Three pounds of fruit, including berries, divided into three meals. Chew very well.

Rice day
3 × 50g rice, brown rice is best, boiled in water without salt; in the morning and in the evening eat with stewed apples or apple purée; at noon, add two tomatoes stewed with herbs.

Raw fruits, grains and vegetables
In the morning, fruit or muesli from your health food shop, at noon and in the evening a salad plate: grated root vegetables, leafy salads, sauerkraut, no mayonnaise. Prepare with a dressing made of oil, lemon and herbs.

Say goodbye to cigarettes, alcohol, coffee and sweets. Don't panic. Just say, 'Bye for now, see you next week,' and mean it.

Read up on what you still want to know about fasting, get in touch with experienced fasters. Start your fasting diary (see example on page 47).

Your mental changeover from eating to fasting has already started. A few thoughts at night may be helpful:

- *I have decided to fast and I know I can do it.*
- *The daily grind is behind me.*
- *At last I have time for myself.*
- *I am comfortable here. I feel at ease.*
- *I have all I need: a comfortable place to stay, some juices, water – and the well stocked pantry inside myself.*
- *I am curious to find out where this journey will take me – I am confident it will be a good journey. Nature is my guide and I can depend on it.*

The first day of fasting

Experience has shown that it is best to start a fast by thoroughly cleansing your intestines. For people who have no problems of elimination, this is relatively easy and only needs a little help. Half a glass of sauerkraut juice, whey or buttermilk taken in the morning helps elimination. However, a great many people tend to be constipated. If you are one of these, you need stronger measures. The following methods of cleansing the intestines have proven effective during a fast. Dissolve 40g (1½ oz) of Glaubersalts in ¾ litres (1½ pints) warm water (30g/1 oz) for small people in ½ litre/1 pint). Drink the solution within 15 minutes. To improve the taste, you may drink some mint herbal tea before and after taking the Glaubersalts solution, to which you may add some lemon juice.

Within the next one to three hours you will experience several spontaneous bowel movements, which may last until the afternoon. So it is wise to remain near a toilet.

If you have a delicate stomach or intestines, you should avoid Glaubersalts. The same is true for very slim people. You should take an enema instead, which will be just as effective. The proper way to do this is explained further on.

Should you feel some light cramps, go to bed and apply a hot water bottle. Make sure your feet are warm. Another hot water bottle will help. Quench your thirst with plenty of water or mint tea.

Women who are used to taking the Pill in the morning should take it about three hours after drinking the Glaubersalts. This precaution is necessary, as the Glaubersalts may empty the stomach prematurely. If an enema is taken, it is not necessary to delay taking the Pill.

The thorough cleansing of the bowel starts the fast. The body switches from 'intake' to 'elimination'. It begins to live on its inner reserves and you will no longer feel hungry. On this first day it is best to stay at home. Lie down when you feel like it, read, relax. Perhaps a walk in the afternoon, but no great physical exertions. Do not take hot baths or use the sauna.

What you can drink

In the morning: 2 cups of herbal tea (camomile, mallow leaf, rosemary or melissa) or a weak black tea with lemon or ginseng tea, perhaps with ½ teaspoon of honey.
In between: Plenty of water or mineral water. Occasionally, suck on a lemon wedge.
Lunch: ¼ litre (½ pint) of homemade vegetable broth. See recipes below for 4 different kinds. Or fresh vegetable juice, water added to make ½ litre (1 pint), or bottled vegetable juice diluted with water. May be taken hot or cold.
Afternoon: 2 cups of fruit tea (rosehip, fennel or apple peel) or mild black tea (not after 4 p.m.) with lemon and/or ½ teaspoon honey if desired.
Evening: ¼ litre (½ pint) fruit juice of your choice, diluted with mineral water, cold or hot, or vegetable juice, or hot vegetable broth (the same as at noon).

Drink very slowly, 'chewing' each mouthful. Savour it! Fasting liquids provide the body with vitamins and minerals, alkaline substances and easily digested carbohydrates, which counterbalance the acidosis occurring during a fast. Drink water and mineral water according to your thirst, more rather than less. Water is an important dissolving and cleansing agent for the detoxified body.

Vegetable and fruit juices are too concentrated on their own and should be diluted with water. If they do not agree with you, you should add a teaspoon of linseed. The gelatinous properties of linseed absorb fruit and vegetable acids.

For people with a delicate stomach, fasting with gruel made of oats, rice or linseed is recommended. (Recipes given on page 31.) Often a mouthful of gruel will settle your stomach, even during the night. A thermos flask will keep the gruel warm and handy.

Recipes

(Please note that 1 litre equals roughly 2 pints)

Potato broth

For 4 servings you will need:

1 litre water
½ lb potatoes
2 carrots
½ leek
¼ stick celery
½ teaspoonful caraway seed
½ teaspoons marjoram
1 pinch of sea salt
1 teaspoonful of vegetarian vegetable paste
1 pinch of freshly ground nutmeg
2 teaspoonsful yeast flakes
4 teaspoonsful chopped parsley

Wash vegetables thoroughly. Do not peel. Add to water. Simmer for 10 to 20 minutes until vegetables are soft. Put through a sieve or use blender, add spices, yeast flakes and parsley.

Carrot broth

For four servings you will need:

1 litre water
½ lb carrots
½ leek
a little celery
1 pinch of sea salt
1 teaspoonful vegetable paste (from the health food shop)
1 pinch grated nutmeg
2 teaspoonsful yeast flakes
4 teaspoonsful chopped parsley

Prepare as above.

Celery broth

For four servings you will need:

1 litre water
½ celery root
some leek and carrot
½ teaspoonful each of caraway and marjoram
1 pinch of sea salt
1 teaspoonful vegetable paste
1 pinch of freshly ground nutmeg
2 teaspoonsful yeast flakes
4 teaspoonsful freshly chopped parsley

Prepare as above. You may also season this soup with basil or lovage.

Tomato broth

For four servings you will need:

1 litre water
1 lb of tomatoes
1 clove of garlic
a little leek, celery or carrot
1 pinch of sea salt
1 teaspoonful vegetable paste
1 pinch of freshly ground nutmeg
2 teaspoonsful yeast flakes
2 teaspoonsful oregano or marjoram

Prepare as above. If desired, you may season this broth with tomato paste.

For sensitive stomachs

Oat gruel

For one serving you will need:

½ litre (1 pint) water
3 tablespoonsful oats

Simmer oats with water for five minutes, pass through a sieve or use a blender. Drink the gruel slowly, one mouthful after the other. If desired, you may season the gruel with a little salt, yeast concentrate, honey, vegetable or fruit juice.

Rice gruel

For one serving you will need:

½ litre (1 pint) water
3 tablespoonsful rice

Prepare as oat gruel.

Linseed gruel

For one serving you will need:

½ litre (1 pint) water
15-20g (½-¾ oz) linseed (Linusit if available)

Simmer linseed for 5 minutes in the water. Use a large pot, as linseed has a tendency to foam. Let stand for five minutes and strain off the gruel. If desired, season the gruel as described above.

The second fasting day

On the second fasting day your body is still getting used to the switchover to your own reserves. You may possibly feel some hunger pangs. Half a glass of water will take care of them. (No appetite depressants!)

It is also possible that your reduced blood pressure has not quite stabilized. You may feel a bit low or experience occasional dizziness. This is quite harmless and a walk in fresh air or some cold water splashed on your face should take care of it. If need be, lie down for a few minutes.

At the beginning of the fasting week, it is not unusual to have a headache or muscular pains. Hot, moist compresses will bring quick relief. Potatoes boiled in their jackets and wrapped in a towel hold the heat for a long time and when applied to the back of the neck, the sacrum or the joints will bring quick relief. A cold Priessnitz compress, (see page 43) an enema, or a footbath will help.

Some people feel depressed, others begin to have doubts about the fast. These feelings will be quickly overcome if you do what usually helps you overcome a psychological 'hangover'. Do not force yourself to do anything you don't really want to do. On the other hand, do not give in too much to your low spirits. And just to be on the safe side, on this second fasting day, give a wide berth to food shops and restaurants. Drink lots of water. If you still experience hunger pangs, void the bowels thoroughly in the morning either by taking an enema or by drinking one scant tablespoon of Glauber or Epsom salts dissolved in a large glass of warm water.

From the third fasting day on

Beginning with the third day of fasting you will be more stable and feel more sure of yourself and more confident. You will experience how well the body has adjusted to living of its inner resources. You are now able to do anything a person who eats normally can do.

At least on the third and fifth day of the fast the intestines should be cleansed by an enema. The bowel in most cases does not continue to function on its own, at least not sufficiently. People who suffer from constipation or stomach or intestinal troubles fast better and with less discomfort if they take an enema every day.

The fasting week at a glance

	What to take	Elimination	Exercise/rest	Hygiene	Experiences
The day before Morning	eg: Fruit and nuts or muesli	Plenty of fibre in the diet to help cleanse the bowels – linseed and wheat bran, and drink plenty of water	Go for a run in the fresh air, then have a rest	Take a bath, relax	Let go of everyday worries
Midday	Raw vegetable salad, potatoes, vegetables, cottage cheese				
Afternoon	One apple/10 hazelnuts				
Evening	Fruit or fruit salad with linseed or wheat bran, 1 yogurt, crispbread, drink plenty of water				
Day 1 of fast Morning	Herb tea Glaubersalts (with lemon) or enema	Prelude to fast: thorough bowel cleansing	Take your usual morning exercise	Sleep as long as you like, making sure feet are warm	Switch from intake to elimination
Mid morning	Sip water occasionally				Keep warm
Midday	Vegetable broth or vegetable cocktail	Help detoxify the liver by lying down	Stay at home	Keep warm	
Afternoon	Herb or fruit tea (with ½ tsp honey)		Afternoon nap, take a short walk	Liver compress	
Evening	Fruit or vegetable juice or vegetable broth			Early to bed	

	What to take	Elimination	Exercise/rest	Hygiene	Experiences
Day 2 of fast Morning	Herb tea (with ½ tsp honey)	Drink more water than usual to flush kidneys and tissues	Stretching exercises, morning walk	Splash cold water on the face. Take an air bath, brush your skin. Keep warm	It's OK to be tired! Relax, feel free from hunger
Mid morning	Sip water occasionally				
Midday	Vegetable broth or vegetable cocktail	If urine is dark, drink more	Afternoon nap	Liver compress	
Afternoon	Herb or fruit tea		Take a walk in the fresh air in the mid afternoon	Make sure hands and feet are warm	
Evening	Fruit juice, vegetable juice or vegetable broth			Do not take a bath or sauna	
Day 3 of fast Morning	Herb tea	To aid bowel elimination, take an enema every second day – if necessary use Epsom or Glauber salts	Morning exercises	Shower, brush your skin and apply oil	Ask yourself 'What does my body need?' 'What does my mind need?'
Mid morning	Sip water occasionally		Satisfy your urge to take exercise – but don't overdo it	Keep warm	
Midday	Tomato broth		Afternoon nap	Liver compress	
Afternoon	Herb or fruit tea				
Evening	Fruit juice, vegetable juice or vegetable broth				
Day 4 of fast Morning	Herb tea	Spontaneous bowel movement? (This is rare)	Keep active: long walks, sport and physical work alternating with rest and relaxation	Walk/run in the dew or snow – brush – shower – oil on skin	Enjoy the fresh morning air
Mid morning	Sip water occasionally				
Midday	Carrot broth	If urine is dark, drink more		Relax lying down	Take sufficient exercise
Afternoon	Herb or fruit tea	Skin odour may have changed, or unpleasant taste in mouth – this is normal		You may take a bath or sauna – allow enough relaxation	Keep your body and limbs warm
Day 5 of fast Morning	Herb tea	Cleanse the intestines: enema, Epsom or Glauber salts	Take enough exercise at your own pace. Don't overdo it	Brush – shower – apply oil	You can be proud of yourself: Go shopping for the return to eating

	What to take	Elimination	Exercise/rest	Hygiene	Experiences
Mid morning	Sip water occasionally			Keep feet warm	
Midday	Celery broth			Liver compress	
Afternoon	Herb or fruit tea			Wind down before bed	
Evening	Fruit juice, vegetable juice, or vegetable broth				
Day 1 of eating Morning	Herb tea	Getting used to eating again – take it slowly	Morning exercises or sport **before** breaking the fast	Cold shower or wash in cold water	Eating today is more important than ever before!
Mid morning	Breaking the fast: one very ripe apple or stewed apple/apple purée	Elimination is still important: eat fibre, drink water	Walks, afternoon nap	Keep warm	Concentrate fully on each meal
Midday	Potato and vegetable soup	Eat fibre, drink water		Liver compress	'Enough is plenty'
Afternoon	Drink as before				
Evening	Tomato or asparagus soup, yogurt with linseed, crispbread Soak dried fruit for tomorrow			If you feel 'bloated' – Priessnitz compress	
Day 2 of eating Morning	Morning drink prunes, bread, butter, cottage cheese	Don't worry if your weight increases – this is normal	You may feel lethargic – go for a walk	Stimulate the circulation – skin brushing and fresh air, shower, relax lying down	Are you 'satisfied' or "full"? You should feel contented
Midmorning	Sip water occasionally				
Midday	Leafy salad	If no spontaneous bowel movement, take linseed and drink water, or wait until tomorrow	Don't overdo things	Don't take a bath or sauna	
Afternoon	Herb tea				
Evening	Grated carrot with linseed, wholemeal bread, butter, cottage cheese				

Chapter 4
Proper fasting made easy

Getting up in the morning

The blood circulation and the muscles function normally, but not as quickly as usual. If you leap out of bed in the morning, you may find yourself back in it in a hurry with dizziness or nausea. Get up differently:

- *While still in bed, yawn and stretch like a cat.*
- *Sit for a moment on the edge of the bed before getting up.*
- *Splash some cold water on your face.*
- *Take a quiet walk in the fresh morning air, breathing through the nose.*

If you want to do a little more for your body or if your blood pressure is low, here are three tips on how to start your day:

The Kneipp method*

Wash your whole body from head to toe with cold water. Do not dry yourself, but get back to bed quickly.

Or, take a short cold shower and get back to bed.

Or, take a hot shower followed by rinsing the arms and the face with cold water, beginning at the finger tips working up to the elbows.

Or, go for a 10-minute run through the wet grass or snow and back to bed.

* Sebastian Kneipp (1821-1897) was a Catholic priest in Bad Wörrishofen, Germany. As a young theology student, Kneipp cured himself of a serious lung disease by bathing in the ice-cold river. He was following the teachings of Dr Siegmund Hahn, who had written a book on hydrotherapy. Kneipp later systematized and enlarged Hahn's theories. Today, in Germany, there are numerous spas that apply Kneipp's treatments.

Five minutes of morning exercises

No competitive sports, but just to wake up your tired limbs, stretch all the muscles, loosen stiff joints, relax a stiff back and get your sluggish circulation moving. Perhaps you will do it to music to cheer you up. In short, the exercises should be relaxed, as if you were doing them for fun.

An air bath at the open window

Massage your whole body, starting with the tips of your toes and fingers with a rough terry cloth towel, a fairly hard brush or a sisal glove. Brush vigorously until you feel completely warm. The whole exercise should take from 5 to 10 minutes. Now your circulation should be stable.

After bathing and brushing, use a skin oil. Your skin will absorb it so readily that you need not worry about staining your clothes.

During the fast, just as at any other time, it is often difficult to get started in the morning. Just follow the above advice and you can overcome this difficulty.

Elimination

During fasting, all 'flood gates' of the body are open. The self-cleansing of the body through cleansing the bowels on the first day of fasting is by no means the end of the process. Through all its orifices and pores, the body rids itself of all wastes that have accumulated over the years.

Elimination through the bowels

Normally the functions of the bowels are the intake of nourishment and the elimination of waste. During the fast, the bowels' only function is elimination. To purge the intestines, an enema should be administered every second day.

This is how you can give yourself an enema. In your bathroom, fill an enema container or a douche bag with one litre of lukewarm water. Run some of the water off into the washbowl or into the toilet to eliminate air bubbles. Clamp the hose or, if there is one, turn the screw at the end of the hose to stop the water from flowing out. Slightly grease the end of the rectal tube. Hang the container or bag from the doorknob, which is just about the right height, position yourself on your knees and elbows on the floor and introduce the rectal tube as deeply as possible into the rectum. Let the water flow in slowly, while you relax your abdomen and breathe quietly. Within 2 to 5 minutes, you will feel the urgent need to use the toilet and eliminate the water and any wastes left in the bowels in two or three bursts.

The enema may seem like an outdated device, but it remains the most effective and gentlest measure for the care of the bowels. It adds considerably to the wellbeing of the faster and brings quick relief from hunger pangs, headaches or muscular aches. It is worthwhile to get used to the enema, for it remains one of the most important home care devices for the whole family to treat fever or other upsets.

If a glass of sauerkraut juice (one cup), whey or buttermilk taken in the morning leads to a bowel movement, then that may suffice.

If you are unable to administer an enema, you should drink two teaspoons of Epsom salts dissolved in a glass of warm water. You may have to find out for yourself what is most effective for you by experimenting. Bear in mind, however, that most of the usual laxatives, including the salts, interfere considerably with the quiet functioning of the bowels.

As long as we fast, the bowels eliminate toxic wastes, even up to 20 days after the end of the fast.

Elimination through the urine

At times the urine may be rather dark and have a strong odour. You should drink more water than your thirst requires. Water is ideal to flush the kidneys and the urinary tract. At times you void a lot of urine and at other times very little. This is normal. You can tell by your weight that there are phases where the body retains water and others where it eliminates it. Don't be discouraged if your weight does not drop.

Never take diuretics! They disturb the wisely regulated balance in your body and only seem to be helping for a day or two.

Voiding through the skin

The rather disagreeable odour given off by the skin during the fast will give you an idea of the poisons that are being eliminated through perspiration and soaked up by your underwear, if it is absorbent. It is best therefore to avoid synthetic fibres.

Fasters will feel the need to wash, bathe and take showers often. Before you take a sauna or a swim, a shower is an absolute necessity. While you are fasting your skin will dry out a little and will need daily care with a good herbal oil, such as Diaderma, or products by Weleda, available in most health food shops.

During fasting, you should avoid skin creams, make-up, and face powder, as such products only clog up your pores and prevent the skin from breathing and eliminating.

Use underarm deodorants sparingly to avoid skin irritations.

Most importantly, look forward to the smooth and delicate skin you will have after the fast!

Exhaling metabolic wastes through the lungs

The air you exhale is full of gaseous metabolic waste which will quickly disappear when you go for a walk. If you remain inside, you will have to air out the room thoroughly. At least once every hour you should open the windows or doors for about five minutes. At night, turn off the heating and sleep with open windows.

Self-cleansing through the mucous membranes of the upper respiratory system

Normally the nose, throat and oesophagus clean themselves. The fresh morning air stimulates you to blow your nose and clear your throat. A few handfuls of cold water splashed on your face has the same effect. The self-cleansing of the mucous membranes is intensified during fasting. It is a good opportunity to heal damage done by smoking. Therefore an absolute break from smoking is necessary during fasting. Chewing gum or peppermints can alleviate the 'empty feeling' in your mouth.

Self-cleansing through the vagina

There is a similar tendency for self-cleansing in the mucous membranes of the vagina. During fasting, there may be more vaginal discharge than usual.

Elimination through the mouth

Your tongue may have a bluish-grey film. Sometimes it may even turn brown or black, depending on the type of poison your body is getting rid of. Your teeth and gums often have a bad-smelling coating. You may have a stale taste in your mouth. Increase dental care. Use a toothbrush on your tongue as well, and rinse your mouth frequently. Or suck on a slice of lemon, several times a day.

Your tonsils are equally involved in the elimination process. If you have a strong unpleasant odour from your mouth, take one teaspoon of fuller's earth in a little water, according to directions. This powdered earth absorbs toxic substances and deodorizes them. You may also chew fresh herbs, such as parsley or dill.

Elimination of emotional waste

There is also such a thing as emotional waste. Do not be afraid of disturbing dreams. Do not fear anger, aggression, depression and other 'negative' emotions. The important thing is to express what worries you. If you are unable to discuss your fears, write them down and look at what you have written at a later time, 'in the light of day'. In any case, you must also come to terms with the emotional waste. You will find a great relief after this coming to terms.

What you can expect to accomplish during the fast

How much fasters can expect to accomplish does not depend as much on the fast, but on their normal performance. There is a full energy supply within; you can do just about everything you usually do. Try it for yourself!

The older person will mostly go for walks. Handicapped people will do what they are able to do. Even someone who does not exercise regularly is perfectly capable of digging the garden, for example, as long as you do not do it too quickly, but calmly and rhythmically.

There are, however, some small differences which you should be aware of. Anything requiring a quick spurt of energy, such as running up the stairs, trying to catch a moving train, playing soccer or skiing can be a problem for fasters. They will do much better at something requiring long-term stamina, such as swimming, hiking, bicycling, rowing, walking up a hill slowly but steadily, or doing gymnastics. What is important is that fasters reach their performance limit daily. Thus they ensure that their fitness is preserved even during the fast. Fitness training with the goal of improving one's physical performance is just as feasible during fasting as at any other time and follows the same rules:

- *daily exercise*
- *exercise all muscle groups*
- *reach your performance limit once or twice daily*
- *start gradually and build up*
- *ensure a harmonious balance between exercise and rest.*

Fitness training increases the muscles while actually reducing weight. Strength and performance follow the law of demand – or of function. The parts of the body being used are not reduced – in fact they are built up with proper training. The properly nourished faster has plenty of protein reserves and only fat is broken down to supply energy.

A faster who stays in bed will lose strength and be as unfit as a person who eats normally but does not move about. Many have this experience when in hospital. People who are lazy lose weight just as active people do but they lose not only fat but also muscle. Then they wonder why their circulation gives them problems and why they feel tired.

Consider the following two examples:

The 54-year-old 10000 metre runner, Schweizer, trained every day of his 50-day fast. On the 49th day of his fast, he ran his best time ever.

A 40-year-old man who was very active in sports fasted for 21 days and lost 24 pounds. He exercised daily, played tennis, swam and hiked for hours. He returned home beautifully fit. A year later, he fasted again, this time with his leg in plaster: he had broken it in an accident. Except for walking a little with the aid of a stick and some exercises in his room, he could do nothing. After 21 days the plaster cast was removed. He had again lost 24 pounds, but he felt weak, had to learn how to walk again and only after six weeks of vigorous training was he back in shape.

The faster is also capable of mental efforts, and creative, artistic pursuits – often with far better results than usual. I remember an 82-year-old who experienced an unusually creative phase during his fast.

An Austrian philosopher claimed that he did his best writing while fasting. I know of painters who experienced a wealth of impressions of colours and shapes during their fast, which they translated into pictures only after the fast had ended; others experienced unusually productive phases.

A faster can treat himself to massages, sunbathing and therapeutic baths and Kneipp treatments (see page 36). Those who regularly enjoy a sauna may do so now, but should restrict themselves to two sessions of 10 minutes each. After leaving the sauna, you should splash cold water on your *face* first, not on your legs!

Resting three times a day

The quickest way to physical and mental wellbeing is to alternate tension and relaxation, effort and rest.

After every exertion, after a bath, sauna or massage or any other therapeutic treatment you should rest. Do not read. Close your eyes, exhale quietly and rest. The metabolism needs the necessary time to accomplish its tasks, it transforms, it builds up and breaks down. It needs time for these processes.

At any rate, you should have an afternoon nap. It is helpful to place a half-filled hot water bottle on your stomach. Even better is a hot moist compress, the so-called liver compress. It supports the liver in its detoxification process. Just by lying down, the blood circulation in the liver is multiplied 40 times. You can rest in your bed, on a sofa or in the grass. The important thing is that you lie down, relax and are warm.

Relaxation

Those who have mastered the art of letting go and relaxing will overcome adversities much faster. During fasting, the body is ready to relax. This is an excellent time to learn the art of relaxation and of concentrating on your own body with the help of various methods, such as autogenic training, yoga, proper breathing or exercises.

Fasting nights

According to an old saying, 'If you fast, you will not sleep. Do not complain. Make use of the time.' However, about half of those who fast have no more trouble sleeping than they normally do. Most sleep soundly, albeit not as long as usual. Many fasters can improve their chances of falling asleep or of sleeping through the night. Here are some simple tips:

Getting ready for bed

Wind down and relax. Let the day come to an end gently. Do not watch exciting television programmes just before going to bed. A short walk is far better. So is sitting quietly in a chair reading a book that you enjoy; listen to music that you love – in short, do something that you know relaxes you. All impressions we absorb continue in our sleep, albeit subconsciously.

Relieve cerebral congestion. The blood congestion after intensive mental effort or heated discussions can be relieved by a walk in the fresh air, by an increasingly warm foot bath, by a few knee bends or sit-ups; or by any physical activity that drains the blood from your head to the muscles.

Avoid cold feet. See the section on 'keeping warm' (page 43) for fast relief.

Open the window. Lack of oxygen may cause bad dreams. Turn off the heating, and sleep with the window open. If you are cold, do not close the window, but put an extra blanket on your bed.

No sleeping pills or pain killers. Avoid all medication that you can possibly do without. If need be, have your usual medication handy on your bedside table. If you are very uncomfortable, take it, but only after having tried all natural means to promote sleep.

If your sleep is disturbed

Your sleep may be disturbed if you feel restless or unwell. You can quickly improve this situation if you pay attention to the following:

A full stomach not only does not like to 'think', it also does not like to sleep. Even during fasting, you may feel distended through intestinal gases or you may be uneasy with cramps, especially during the post-fasting period. A Priessnitz compress will bring quick relief. Dip one third of a linen towel into cold water, wring it out and fold it in such a way that there are two dry parts and one wet part. Put the cold, wet part over your stomach with the dry parts around your back. Put a dry, folded terry cloth towel on top of the compress, which will become agreeably warm within a short time.

If you toss and turn in your bed or get up frequently, you should wash from head to toe with cold water, using a washcloth, not the shower. Get back to bed without drying yourself. You will be surprised how effective this simple remedy will prove, even if, possibly, you sleep less deeply and for a shorter time during fasting. Remember the motto of this chapter: 'Do not complain'. So if you wake up before your usual time, don't grumble. Just accept your wakefulness. 'Make use of the time'. Enjoy the silence of the night or of daybreak. If you think about your job, or your family, accept those thoughts. Do not shy away from thinking about yourself for once. Have a pad and pencil ready and jot down some of your thoughts. Many people have found the key to self-discovery or the long-sought-after solution to their problems during such fasting nights. Or why not read a bit? Often, we do not find time to read during our working days.

The next morning, you will realize that you are not even tired. Only those who cannot accept the waking hours and are angry about lying awake will feel tired in the morning. It is a known fact that fasters can manage with five or six hours of sleep, especially if they take the recommended breaks during the day.

Keeping warm

Do not be surprised if your hands and feet are often cold while fasting. The 'inner

43

stove' can produce the same amount of heat from layers of fat as it can from food, but during a fast it always switches to 'low burn'. It is as if the body had to manage its reserves carefully.

This is how you can remedy the problem

Clothing should be light, but warm.

Choose natural, warm and absorbent fibres such as cotton, lawn and wool; do not wear synthetics. Wear shoes whose inner soles are made of cork or leather; in the summer wear light sandals or wooden clogs.

Exercise produces warmth. Hot drinks make one more comfortable than cold drinks. Use hot liver compresses in the morning and again at night. Put a hot water bottle on your feet as soon as they feel cold. A hot footbath is simple: any bucket or plastic basin will do. If you feel thoroughly chilled or even just cold, a hot foot bath in which you make the water increasingly warm is the best preventive measure against colds. Lukewarm water, not hot, is poured into a bucket or basin up to the calves. Hot water is added in intervals to ensure that the feet get a constant new supply of warmth. In 15 to 20 minutes, the whole body is warm. Then quickly apply a little cold water and put yourself into warm socks or into bed. During a fast, the body cools off quicker after a bath or swimming. Shorten your swimming time a little and remember to warm up properly afterwards.

Different ways fasting can affect you

Eyesight. You may note that your eyesight diminishes and print becomes unclear. Eye pressure is slightly reduced during fasting. Do not worry, it rights itself very quickly and after a fast your eyesight is usually improved. However, be careful while driving a car: ability to concentrate and to react may be reduced.

Understanding. You may read something once, twice and fail to understand what you have read even after the third try. You may have difficulty grasping a point. Do not be disturbed. This problem too will not last more than a couple of days.

Remembering. You may forget very quickly what has just been said. You may forget commitments you have made or even your own telephone number. You may be slower to find the right expression. Do not be surprised. Even your brain needs a break now and then. It is a sign of turning off after previous overexertion.

Sexual Potency. There may be a temporary change, an increase or decrease. After the fast, it will be more balanced, more normal.

Menstruation. It may be delayed, be heavier or lighter. Here too, it will resume its normal pattern after the fast.

Wellbeing while fasting

After the first day or two, most fasters feel relieved, unburdened and very well. They have gained confidence in fasting, and their surprise at how well they feel turns to joy, the joy of discovering new wellbeing.

Low points during the fast

Of course, life is not all a bed of roses when you fast. There will be some low points, particularly in the morning or at particular times of the day: 'I feel tired; I'm bored; I feel a bit dizzy and sluggish. What am I going to do now? Shall I pull myself together or do I let myself go?' Do both!

Whether you feel let down or listless, pull yourself together first of all. This will in most cases get you over your low point and at the same time cure your lethargy. Take a walk in the fresh air for about ten minutes and you will quickly feel better.

If the let-down feeling persists despite the walk, and despite trying to take part in some sports or other activities, then it is time to let yourself go. It is quite right to retire to your own room, lie down, to read or to sleep.

Pulling yourself together is especially important for people who have a tendency to be sluggish or overweight. The extra pounds often spoil your fun in exercising. And lazy people have let themselves go so often, that they are now completely out of shape. The day will come where the lethargy and the handicaps are overcome and exercise begins to be enjoyable and in the end becomes a felt need. Until that day, remember, don't let yourself go. Pull yourself together!

For people whose blood pressure is below normal (below 100/60) fasting is generally slightly more difficult than for others. They may experience some weakness, dizziness and inability to concentrate. Their circulation will need support:

- *Pay particular attention to the section on getting up in the morning.*
- *Black tea with ½ teaspoon honey taken in the morning and after the liver compress at noon. This is best taken while still lying down. Ginseng tea is equally effective.*
- *Exercise is absolutely necessary to stabilize the circulation – but it has to be started slowly.*

Everybody should walk or hike – at a reasonable speed – in order to prevent low points during fasting.

Crises during fasting

Crises due to fasting rarely occur during a short fast. They happen more frequently during a long fast of 20 days or more and affect sick people more readily than healthy fasters. They come on out of the blue. Fasters feel down, aggravated or depressed. Old ailments flare up. They feel sick – as if they had flu. Fasting crises are healing crises. They are the days or hours during which the body is eliminating most intensively the waste and toxic substances which enter the circulatory system. As soon as all these toxins are expelled from the body, the crisis is over as completely as if it had never happened. When such a crisis occurs, the body is fully occupied and needs to be managed.

- *Bed rest, warmth and an enema are very beneficial.*
- *Take plenty of tea or water.*
- *A glass of buttermilk will work wonders.*
- *During a crisis it would be wrong to force yourself to any activity or to break the fast.*

Tips for fasting during working days

- *Allow extra time for your morning toilette and exercises. That means getting up earlier.*
- *Allow plenty of time to get to work. Avoid rushing. Leave the car at home. Use a bus or tram and get off one stop earlier than usual and walk the rest of the way. Use the stairs instead of the lift – lots of exercise and fresh air are important. Use your lunch hour to go for a walk or have a nap in your chair.*
- *Remember your changed body odour and mouth odour: rinse your mouth frequently with clear water with a few drops of mouthwash added; drink some mint tea without sugar.*
- *After working hours lose yourself in your own personal atmosphere and do all the things others do during their holiday. Go to bed early. Get rid of callers and curious friends. Refuse invitations to go out.*
- *Meet regularly with your fellow fasters or exchange your experiences on the telephone.*

Fasting balance sheet – Summary of complaints

It pays to keep an exact record of your fasting experience. Keep a diary of your diet, the elimination of waste, your physical and mental state, your physical and mental activities. Establish a fasting balance sheet.

Write down all major or minor complaints you have before you begin your fast – and note what has remained after your fast. Determine the results of your week of fasting.

Weight loss

Let us take an example: A man and a woman fast because of moderate overweight.

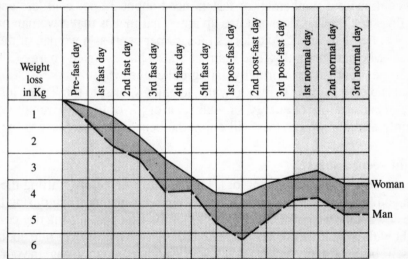

Weight lost during 1-week fast
Example 1: Woman, 40, 160cm, starting weight 65kg.
Example 2: Man, 40, 175cm, starting weight 80kg.

The woman's curve shows an evenly downward, then upward, curve. The man's curve goes down on the first and third day of the fast and shows a much steeper climb on the second and third day after the return to normal eating. This is typical for people whose tissues retain more salt and water. On the fourth day of fasting, the man's weight loss was zero. His body had retained the water. This is perfectly normal;

further salt deposits in the body are dissolved and eliminated via the kidneys the next day. There is no need for concern if your weight remains stationary for days at a time. The real loss of weight in one week of fasting can be noticed on the morning of the first day *after* the fast. The woman lost three kilos (6½ pounds) and the man lost four (9 pounds). For both of them, this represents a normal and average loss of weight. The curve shows the loss of fatty tissue and of water and salt. The curve is not the same for all people and is affected by various factors such as weather, time and medications.

The woman lost about 1.8kg (4 pounds) of fatty tissue during the week's fast, the man lost about 2.5kg (4½ pounds). One kilogram of fatty tissue provides 6000 calories. One can therefore work out that burning up fatty tissue by the woman provided 1500 calories daily of energy, while the man used daily 2100 calories.

To continue our mathematics: fasters need about 30 per cent less energy, since their digestive process does not use up any. That means that a woman has as much energy at her disposal (1500 calories plus 30 per cent) as a woman of the same size and age who eats normally. The man who fasts has as much energy (2100 calories plus 30 per cent) as his normally eating colleague whose intake is 3000 calories.

That is plenty in order to live, to work, to enjoy sports, to think. The loss of weight does not cause a loss of energy, of vitality or of joy of living! Even those who have had only a minor weight loss will enjoy the benefits of their fast to the fullest.

Weight record sheet

Note the course of your weight loss. On the morning before starting the fast, write down your starting weight. Then weigh yourself every morning during the fast and write down your weight. On the morning of the first post-fasting day compare your weight with what it was when you started the fast. Make a firm rule about weighing yourself; be consistent. Always check your weight in the morning, in your nightgown or pyjamas, after voiding the night urine. Or always in the morning after having moved your bowels, always naked. Keep checking your weight in the following months and weeks. Living with the scales is the surest way to keep your weight. Place the scales where you cannot overlook them, and keep your balance sheet and a pencil handy.

Win by losing

Does this sound paradoxical? Let me resume what we have said in the preceding sections. The fasting organism draws vitality and warmth from the energy supply which is fat, and nutrients from stored proteins. It is interesting to note that the body does not burn up just any kind of fat or use up just any kind of proteins. It rids itself of the following substances and in the exact order given:

- *anything that burdens the body*
- *anything the body does not need*
- *anything that disturbs the body*
- *anything that makes the body ill*

Not only do we become ill from the overconsumption of fats and carbohydrates, but also from an oversupply of proteins. This has been proven by recent capillary biology research. Excess protein builds up along the walls of the smallest blood vessels (capillaries), which are found in all organs. These deposits, of which you will be quite unaware yourself, are regarded as the forerunner of many diseases, which may show themselves only years later. This is true of all diseases affecting the metabolism, as well as of most forms of heart disease, and circulatory troubles that may lead to heart attacks and strokes. It is also true for the most common forms of joint rheumatism and non-articular rheumatism, to name but a few examples.

We can protect ourselves against these dangers by ridding our bodies of excess proteins from time to time (such as during a fast) and furthermore to learn not to overload our system with proteins. Therefore fasting and sensible nutrition go hand in hand.

Detoxification is part of the cleansing process that takes place during a fast. Toxins are absorbed by fat and proteins and stored in the soft tissues. When fat and proteins are broken down during the fast, the toxins can be eliminated through the bowels, the kidneys and the skin.

By now you will readily see why we do not want to enrich fasting drinks with protein or use special protein drinks. Doing so would hinder the process of purification and destroy the chances for healing. This does not apply to obese people on a long-term fast (over 30 days and only in a clinic), where loss of weight is more important than detoxification, or to elderly people. In these cases the addition of protein may well be necessary. The body never rids itself of:

- *anything vitally essential, for example heart or muscles*
- *functioning parts of the body, active organs*
- *control devices.*

These natural laws, which are programmed within the human body, are the key to the secret of fasting. We may have full confidence in the reliability of our body.

Improved health

The loss of weight will result in many beneficial changes in the body. It relieves the knee joints, feet, spinal discs, in short, all supporting elements of the body. It relieves the heart which can now pump with less effort and more strongly. Breathing becomes easier, the lungs can absorb more oxygen and blood circulation carries it to the tissues more quickly. Elevated blood pressure sinks to a normal level. While low blood pressure can temporarily cause some tiredness and dizziness, it will soon rise to the normal level. Temporarily elevated blood sugar will get back to normal within the first five days of the fast, but it will never sink below normal. [**Note: Diabetics requiring medication must fast only in a clinic.**]

Too high a concentration of blood fats (cholesterol, triglycerides and others) is reduced daily during the fast. As soon as the blood fat level is normal, fat deposits are broken down in the liver, in the blood vessels and in all other organs where fat deposits are present. Thus fat not only disappears on the outside of the body, but on the inside as well. This is really the beginning of therapeutic fasting.

Even if laboratory tests show that the levels of fat in the liver are slightly above normal, you may be sure that these levels will be improved after as little as five fasting days, if, of course, you really do not drink even one drop of alcohol. People with liver disease should only fast in a clinic. To sum up the results of fasting, we can say that the tendency of these levels, measurable by laboratory tests, to return to normal corresponds to the body's tendency to correct itself (homoeostasis).

Special attention should be paid to any rise in uric acid levels during fasting. Such a rise indicates that considerable breaking down and changing of cells is occurring. Only a few people are bothered by this problem. If you know that you have too high a level of uric acid over a considerable period of time, you should observe the following rules: Drink a lot of liquid (preferably water); two to three lemons a day, squeezed for juice or else cut into wedges for sucking; no alcohol of any kind (not allowed during the fast in any case). It is especially important that the process of eliminating body waste functions well. Patients who are on medication to reduce uric acid levels because of gout should continue taking this medication while fasting. This is best done in a clinic. Eventually the uric acid in the blood will be reduced, but only after five to six days of fasting.

To gradually reduce weight at the same time as exercising the body does a great deal to improve one's health. The loss of each kilo reduces risk factors. Each day of fast cleanses the body. In short, we add healthy and enjoyable years to our lives.

Beauty treatment from within

Time and time again a physician observing a fast is impressed to see how the face of a faster changes. Some examples: a ruddy, bloated 'moon face', covered with red blotches (which the layman may consider healthy), begins to improve and the complexion starts to return to normal after as little as five days of fasting. Dull eyes become clear again and a wavering gaze grows steady. The grey skin of the smoker becomes lighter and fresh-looking. The spongy, large-pored skin of the alcoholic tightens and the redness disappears. The facial expression becomes more self-confident. The tired, resigned and pale face caused by exhaustion turns inward at first and becomes still. But then it fills out, becomes fresh and smooth. The eyes begin to shine; the tautness and elasticity of the skin is striking. Impurities have disappeared, and lines are smoothed out. In the course of one's life, the fibres of the skin and the subcutaneous connecting fibres lose their elasticity. The fibrous structures become thick and stiff, because of the deposits of water, salt and endogenous wastes. This congested tissue can be quite painful if you pinch it (cellulitis).

A purifying fast, combined with exercise and alternately hot and cold showers, brushing to stimulate the blood circulation followed by an application of oil, are infinitely more effective than any beauty treatment from the outside. In a short time you will be able to rejuvenate the connective tissue, to tighten it and to eliminate the pain. When you lose weight, you often fear that you will become flabby. This may happen during fasting; however, during the post-fasting period all tissues are tightened, even the inner organs. After a long fast many people report that they feel five years younger.

The detoxified body becomes taut

How your partner can help

It does not matter whether a couple fasts together or whether just one of you does.

What matters is that both are aware of the basic principles:

To fast means to retreat into yourself; to listen to your body's own rhythm and to act according to the demands of your body and not to the demands or expectations of your partner.

Fasters interrupt their usual habits. They live by different rules. Let go of one another temporarily: you will find each other again with a clearer mind and body.

- *Both of you should become informed about fasting. Read this Guide together.*
- *Make a joint decision about when to start the fast.*
- *Agree on where to fast, when to eat and how to spend your leisure time; schedule your rest.*
- *Change your sleeping habits; separate rooms are recommended because of body odours during fasting and the varying need for fresh air. It will also allow each of the partners to turn on the light, to get up and read, etc. without disturbing the other.*
- *Your sex life may change, but not necessarily. Accept any changes in your partner.*
- *Respect your partner's desire for rest.*
- *Special attention must be paid to hygiene – because of the changed body emanations.*
- *Mood changes are normal during fasting. Accept such changes in your partner. Do not complain if your partner retires more often from your company.*
- *Naturally you should do you best to help your partner resist the temptation to eat, smoke or drink alcohol.*

Temptations overcome

You would not be human if fasting was not full of temptation. 'Just one little bite!' or 'surely an apple can't hurt you.' No, of course an apple cannot really hurt. But each little bit – of whatever it may be – endangers your fast, for it stimulates the appetite. If you stimulate your digestive juices, you must not be surprised if they ask for something to digest! Consequently it is truly easier not to eat at all. Experienced fasters are aware of that fact.

'How about a cup of coffee – that doesn't have any calories. Or some ice cream – that does have a lot of calories but you don't need to chew it.'

Coffee and ice cream are great stimulants for the stomach juices. Therefore they can provoke as much hunger as any other food.

What is truly dangerous is to succumb to the temptation to eat a complete meal – maybe consisting of soup, meat course and desert. Such a slip could have serious consequences – ranging from stomach cramps to a collapse of the circulatory system.

A firm renunciation also has a deeper meaning: overcoming temptation makes one strong. Fears and temptations that one manages to overcome result in maturity and inner growth.

While it is better not to go into town during the first days of fasting or to stop at bakeries or butcher shops, you will be able to do so with surprising ease a little later on. You will be able to sit in a restaurant and order a mint tea or a glass of hot lemonade without sugar or a freshly squeezed orange juice while watching others eat – without feeling hunger pangs yourself.

You will return home very proud of yourself, fortified by a new self-esteem.

How serious is your craving for a cigarette, for alcohol? During a fast you can really tell whether smoking and drinking had been only a habit which you can get away from, or if the dependence on tobacco or alcohol has in fact become an addiction.

A break from smoking and drinking while fasting is not only necessary for your health, but it also answers the question of whether or not you are the master or the slave of your habits.

Here too the principle is to say a clear and firm 'NO' at the beginning of the fasting week. A lot of small, weak 'Nos' later on would just be unnecessary torture.

At the end of your fast, you will have gained so much confidence that you are capable of much more important decisions. For example, why not continue to forego these harmful habits?

Fasting means renunciation and your fasting period gives you a chance to learn to do without. You will learn that in the end 'doing without' is to your benefit. In short, fasting may teach you one of the best human talents, namely to be content with little.

Continuing the fast

Remember that this book is aimed at healthy people. Should you have doubts whether or not to continue the fast, you should discuss the matter with your own doctor.

Do not be afraid to continue the fast as long as you feel well, find that fasting agrees with you and that you have some more weight to lose – in other words if all the prerequisites for fasting on your own are there. A sure sign that you may continue the fast is if your usual work performance remains steady, or better yet, if it improves.

It is of course best to be supervised by a physician experienced in fasting.

Starting with the third week, you will need supplements of vitamins and minerals, since the reserves of these substances in your own body will be exhausted.

You will have to allow extra time for the period in which you return to normal eating, as described on page 56. This period should be at least one-quarter, better yet one-third, of the time period during which you fasted. The rules for the return to normal eating patterns are few but important:

- *eat sparingly*
- *eat simply*
- *eat wholesome food*
- *do not eat hard-to-digest food: no meat, perhaps small helpings of fish, no cold meats or sausages, no hard cheeses, no fried foods*

Fasting: change in nutrition

Learning how to eat properly is often more difficult than fasting. Perhaps it would be best to undertake a short fast three times a year and after these fasts, practise moderate, disciplined eating. You will lose weight gradually and it will be easier for you to maintain your weight.

How often is it safe to fast?

If you eat wholesome food and are in good health but somewhat overweight, you may fast as often as once a month. Why not fast one week, then eat for three weeks? Your body will get used to that rhythm. What makes the difference is that each return to normal eating patterns provides the incentive to change your diet to high quality, wholesome foods.

Many people have made it a rule to detoxify once a year. Others embark on a religiously motivated fast in Lent and during Advent; they experience the physical cleansing together with spiritual renewal.

Fasting in one way or the other should become part of your life. It is good to establish a pattern.

Chapter 5
Breaking the fast –
return to normal eating patterns

Shopping for the first two days of normal eating

Go shopping on the fifth day of fasting. It will be fun to handle food without being dependent on it. For one person, you will need:

1 lb of ripe apples, unsprayed (or well-rinsed)
1 packet each of potato, tomato or asparagus soup, butter, cottage cheese, cream cheese (20% fat)
2 tubs of natural yoghurt
1 packet of rye crispbread, wholemeal or linseed bread,
½ lb of dried prunes or figs
1 bottle of whey or sauerkraut juice.

If you do your own cooking, you will also need salad greens, tomatoes, potatoes and the necessary ingredients for preparing them. Should you be able to obtain organically grown vegetables you will enjoy them more – fasting refines the taste buds, and your food will be healthier.

If you are obliged to eat out, choose whatever comes closest to the menus recommended for the return to normal eating.

Switching over from fasting to eating

The writer George Bernard Shaw, an experienced faster, said: 'Any fool can fast, but only a wise man can break the fast properly.'

Why should it be so complicated? The return to normal eating signifies the rebuilding of the daily functioning of the metabolism and the digestion. The body switches from eating to fasting more quickly than from fasting to eating. The organism has stopped the flow of digestive juices. Now it has to start them up again. This does not happen all of a sudden, but gradually. Therefore the return to eating is a vital part of the fasting process. It needs as much attention, time and rest as fasting itself. In order to ensure a smooth transition, you should observe the following rules:

Three rules for proper eating

Take your time
Do not look at the clock. Eat without hurrying – this is the most important appointment you have today.

Chew well
Digestion begins in the mouth. Each bite should be chewed 35 times until it is liquefied. Gulping down your food is harmful.

Eat in silence
It is the only way to enjoy your food, to satisfy your hunger and to leave the table content. All your attention should focus on the meal – as if you were going to pass a test to see if you know how to eat properly.

The days of returning to normal eating patterns are a critical time for coming to terms with old eating and drinking habits. Fasting interrupted them and you can now throw them overboard if you have come to the conclusion that they were wrong.

To the basic conclusion you will reach on fasting – 'I feel and function very well even without food' – you can now add the lesson you will learn during the return to normal eating: *I need a lot less food than I used to.* This is an opportune time to practise new eating habits, based on the experience you have had.

Diet plan for the return to normal eating

First day after the fast

In the morning: Tea (herbal tea or weak black tea)
Mid morning: Breaking the fast: 1 very ripe or stewed apple
Noon: 1 bowl of potato and vegetable soup (see below)
Afternoon: Fruit tea
Evening: Tomato soup, buttermilk with one teaspoonful of linseed, 1 slice of rye crispbread.

Recipes

(Please note that one litre corresponds to roughly 2 pints, ¼ litre is about 1 cup)

Potato & Vegetable Soup

(Sufficient for one serving)

> *1 small potato, about 60g (2 oz)*
> *one piece each of carrot, leek and celery*
> *¼ litre (½ pint) water*
> *1 pinch each of freshly ground nutmeg and marjoram*
> *½ teaspoonful yeast flakes*
> *1 teaspoonful vegetable paste*
> *1 teaspoonful fresh chopped parsley*

Peel or scrape vegetables and cut into fine strips. Simmer in the water for about 15 minutes with the pot covered. Take off the stove, add spices. If desired pass through a blender. Sprinkle with chopped parsley.

Tomato Soup

(Sufficient for one serving)

> *250g (8 oz) ripe tomatoes*
> *½ onion*
> *1 teaspoonful oil*
> *¼ litre (½ pint) water*
> *1 teaspoonful vegetable paste*
> *1 pinch each of sea salt, freshly ground white pepper and dried thyme*
> *½ teaspoonful yeast flakes*
> *1 teaspoonful tomato purée*
> *1 teaspoonful fresh chopped parsley or chives*

Wash tomatoes, remove stems and chop. Peel and chop onion. Heat the oil, add tomatoes and onions and cook for about 10 minutes. Pass through a sieve or blender. Bring the water to a boil, add the cooked tomatoes, the vegetable paste, tomato purée and yeast flakes. Sprinkle with parsley or chives.

For tomorrow:
Soak two prunes or figs in half a cup of water and let stand overnight.

Second day

1 glass sauerkraut juice or whey.

Morning: Prunes or figs, 'shredded wheat soup'.

For big appetites add 50g (1¾ oz) cottage cheese with herbs, 2 slices of rye crispbread.

Mid-morning: Drink mineral water.

Noon: Leafy salad, potatoes boiled in their jackets, steamed carrots, yoghurt sweetened with buckthorn syrup, and one teaspoonful of linseed added.

Afternoon: Grated carrots, vegetable or grain soup, yoghurt with linseed, 1 slice of rye crispbread.

Shredded wheat soup

(Sufficient for one serving)

> *2 tablespoonsful finely shredded wheat*
> *¼ litre (½ pint) water*
> *1 pinch sea salt*
> *1 tablespoonful chopped fresh herbs such as parsley or chives*

Heat the shredded wheat in a pan without browning it. Add water and let come to the boil. Turn off heat and allow to swell for about 10 minutes, strain off soup if you like. Season with salt and herbs.

Leafy salad

(Sufficient for one serving)

> *¼ head of lettuce*
> *1 pinch each of sea salt and freshly ground pepper*
> *½ teaspoonful cider vinegar or lemon*
> *1 teaspoonful sunflower oil*
> *1 teaspoonful chopped chives*

Wash well and tear leaves, dry in salad spinner. Prepare a dressing of oil, vinegar or lemon juice, salt and pepper. Sprinkle with chives.

Potatoes in their jackets

(Sufficient for one serving)

3 small potatoes
some caraway seeds

Scrub potatoes well under running water, boil with the caraway seeds for 20 to 25 minutes.

Steamed carrots

(Sufficient for one serving)

100g (3½ oz) carrots
3 tablespoonsful water or vegetable stock
1 pinch each of sea salt and freshly ground nutmeg
1 teaspoonful sunflower oil
1 teaspoonful chopped parsley

Scrub carrots under running water and cut into thin slices. Bring water or vegetable stock to the boil, add carrot slices and simmer for about 10 minutes. Take off the heat, add oil, season with salt and pepper and sprinkle with parsley.

Yoghurt with buckthorn syrup and linseed

(Sufficient for one serving)

one container of natural yoghurt
1 teaspoonful buckthorn syrup sweetened with honey
1 heaped teaspoonful linseed

Put yoghurt in a dessert bowl, season with syrup and sprinkle with linseed.

Freshly grated carrots

(Sufficient for one serving)

2 tablespoonsful sour cream
1-2 teaspoonsful lemon juice
a few sprigs of lemon balm
100g (3½ oz) carrots
½ apple
1 salad leaf

Prepare a dressing from the sour cream and the lemon. Scrub carrots under running water, and grate very finely. Add to the dressing. Wash apple, core and grate into the dressing. Serve on lettuce leaf.

Vegetable and grain soup

(Sufficient for one serving)

½ of a small onion
1 teaspoonful olive oil
1 tablespoonful shredded wheat
¼ litre (½ pint) water or vegetable stock
50g (1¾ oz) celery
1 pinch each of lovage and sea salt
1 teaspoonful chopped parsley

Peel and chop onions and brown them slightly in the oil, add shredded wheat and brown slightly. Add water or vegetable stock and simmer for about 10 minutes. Scrub celery and grate very finely. Season soup with salt and lovage, add parsley and grated celery.

Yoghurt with linseed

Mix three tablespoonsful of natural yoghurt with buckthorn syrup sweetened with honey, add a heaped tablespoon of linseed. Eat with one slice of rye crispbread.

After the third day of returning to normal eating the course is set for proper nutrition after the fast – a chance to correct the mistakes you made in your diet in the past. There is hardly a better opportunity to change your eating habits than after fasting.

For tomorrow: soak 1 teaspoonful of raisins for your muesli.

Third day

Fresh vegetables – for all those who enjoy them and want to continue losing weight (800 Calories).

Morning: Herbal tea, later Birchermuesli
Mid morning: Fruit of your choice
Noon: Large fresh vegetable salad (leaf salad and beetroot with horseradish dressing) and one boiled potato
Afternoon: One apple and 12 hazelnuts (filberts) or 4 walnuts
Evening: Large salad plate of your favourite salads or uncooked vegetables.
Important: Raw vegetables must be prepared just before they are eaten, and they should be very well chewed during eating.

Birchermuesli

(Sufficient for one serving)

1 cup of milk or yoghurt
1 small apple
2 teaspoonsful oat flakes
1 teaspoonful grated nuts
1 teaspoonful of honey or raisins which have been soaked
1 teaspoonful lemon juice

Pour milk or yoghurt into a glass bowl, wash and core apple, grate or cut into small pieces. Add oat flakes, nuts and mix well. Stir in honey or the soaked and drained raisins. Season with lemon juice.

Note: You may vary your muesli by using various kinds of fruit, different cereals and nuts.

Some basic rules for the post-fasting period

Morning: Birchermuesli or fresh grain soup.
Noon: Salad or raw vegetables eaten *before* the meal.
Evening: Eat sparingly and not too late.

Your body during the post-fasting period

One third of the whole fasting period should be devoted to a period of rebuilding, a return to normal eating. This post-fasting period is even more important than the fasting period itself. It requires the same basic elements such as rest, comfort and time.

Digestive juices

No digestive juices are produced while you fast. During the post-fasting period digestive juices are first produced in small quantities which increase gradually. Your stomach will tell you how fast and in what quantity your digestive juices flow. Now is the time not to eat everything that is put in front of you. Make a decision at each and every meal how much food will agree with you.

The body cleansed by fasting sends signals. You will be more aware of them than in the past.

> '*I am satisfied*' means: I have had enough to eat. I am no longer hungry. This is all I need. I will stop here and leave the rest.
>
> '*I am full*' means: My stomach is completely full. I have eaten more than I can digest. Half-digested food causes problems such as intestinal gases and a bloated stomach.
>
> '*I can't eat any more*' means: I have stretched my stomach. I cannot digest properly.

The production of digestive juices is stimulated by: proper chewing, raw foods, fruit acids (raw apple), lactic acids (sour milk and yoghurt), herbal spices.

The production of digestive juices is blocked by haste, stress, cold feet, anger, ice cold foods or drinks.

The circulatory system

About one-third of the energy expended by the circulatory system is needed to handle digestion. This third of the total energy available was not needed during fasting. You should therefore not be surprised if your efficiency falls off slightly during the first two days of the post-fasting period. It is possible that you tire more easily, feel a certain emptiness in your head and even experience some dizziness. Especially after a meal, a considerable amount of blood is drawn to the abdominal area and is therefore not available to the head or muscles.

You can remedy this situation by resting after every meal, and by taking your afternoon nap in bed. Before getting up, stretch your muscles, tighten them and then relax. Do not exert yourself unnecessarily.

Filling up

Our body, slightly dehydrated through the fast, absorbs up to one litre (1¾ pints) of water in three post-fasting days. You can tell by your scales (see section on loss of weight and weight balance, page 47.) The water is needed for the flow of the digestive juices and the mucous membranes. It also helps the blood circulation, which from the third day on will be back to normal and completely stable. Water tightens all the inner cells, as you can tell by your smooth facial skin and the disappearance of small wrinkles. To reduce this water by taking diuretics is not sensible, indeed it is dangerous. Therefore you should continue to drink more than your thirst requires. Your bowels should have enough liquids to ensure a soft stool.

The intestines

The bowels will only function on their own when they are filled. So don't be impatient! *Fillers and softeners* are:

- *linseed, 2 teaspoons with every meal, or bran;*
- *raw foods and vegetables;*
- *wholemeal bread, whole grain flakes, wheat bran.*

The first spontaneous bowel movement usually happens on the second day, some-times not until the third. Do not take laxatives! Sometimes the rectum has retained some dried faeces from the fast. You can feel the bowel moving, but the anus does not want to open. It is sufficient to use a remedy that does not interfere with the whole digestive tract, but treats only the rectum:

- *100ml (⅛ pint) warm water administered with a rubber syringe;*
- *a small enema with ½ litre (1 pint) water;*
- *glycerine suppositories (available in drug stores or pharmacies).*

The last full enema should have been taken on the last fasting day or on the first post-fasting day. Cleansing the rectum is necessary until elimination is satisfactory. During the following day, elimination should function normally. People who tend to be constipated should observe some basic rules:

To promote normal bowel movements

- *Drink one glass of water every morning on an empty stomach (nervous people should drink it warm, otherwise cold);*
- *soaked prunes or figs or muesli in the morning;*
- *thoroughly chewed food that contains plenty of fibre (linseed, raw fruit and vegetables, wholemeal bread, whole grain cereals, wheat bran);*
- *exercise of any kind;*
- *allow time for your bowel movement and relax.*

Factors which interfere with normal elimination

- *getting up late;*
- *lack of exercise, sedentary job without compensating exercises or walks;*
- *stress, pressures of deadlines;*
- *cold hands or feet;*
- *impatient pressing during a bowel movement.*

Flatulence

People who are easily cold should use a warm, moist compress on their abdomen, and a hot water bottle. People who tend to be too hot, use a cold Priessnitz compress (see page 43). An infusion made with caraway and fennel seeds is also helpful. Use natural means to eliminate, such as the enema or glycerine suppositories. Note that every bite you have not chewed well may cause flatulence. If you eat too quickly, air is swallowed along with the food.

After-effects of fasting

It is possible that during the first two post-fasting days, old complaints you suffered from before fasting may recur. This strange behaviour of your body may cause quite a disappointment, but it is definitely not a sign that the fast has been unsuccessful. The next day you are likely to feel perfectly well and the complaints give way to increased wellbeing.

The question of what you have really achieved by fasting can only be answered at the end of the post-fasting period. Therefore you should not draw up your list of complaints too early.

Mistakes made during the post-fasting period

The vitality and ability to enjoy yourself that you gained during the fast often tempt you to go off the straight and narrow as early as the third or fourth post-fasting day.

As an example of what can happen, let us use the account given to me by a group of people who had finished their fast.

Three men and two women celebrated the end of their fast. After the post-fasting evening meal, they went to a good restaurant.

Mr W. ordered the steak he had been dreaming about while he fasted. He ate it without leaving the tiniest morsel. Three hours later he called the doctor. 'I felt as if I wanted to die but couldn't,' he later told me. He had atrocious stomach cramps and only after having vomited up his half-digested dinner did he sink back into his bed, white as a sheet and perspiring profusely. *Decomposed undigested protein acts like poison.*

Mrs S. ate her way through the whole menu, finishing with ice cream topped with whipped cream. Her distended stomach told her that all this had not agreed with her. Worse was to come. The next morning, the scales registered a gain of 1.3 kilograms (3 pounds). Three days of fasting down the drain!

Mr A. enjoyed the good wine, to the point where his friends had to get him home and into bed. Laboratory tests showed what had happened. His liver had been damaged by his alcohol consumption. *Just as during the fast, the liver has to be managed during the post-fasting period. The tolerance of alcohol is greatly diminished.* Even the smallest quantity can make you drunk and damage the liver cells.

Mrs K. had dined modestly and then taken a cup of coffee. She thought the night would never end. She was wide awake. 'But coffee never used to keep me from sleeping.' *The nervous system now reacts more strongly* to coffee as well as to medications.

Mr N. had ordered fish. He did not want very much of it and left about half. He had no problems. Only . . . he had intended to observe the post-fasting period carefully. Why had he let himself be talked into going to a restaurant?

During the fast the group had been in good spirits and had enjoyed themselves. Why was the going-away party so dull? They had managed to have a good time when they had only water to drink. Perhaps they could not get into the mood since food was so much the centre of attention?

The post-fasting period makes us more aware of any behaviour problems we habitually experience. Let us recall once again the words of George Bernard Shaw: 'Any fool can fast, but only the wise man knows how to break the fast.'

The post-fasting period is the most important phase of the fast as a whole. It requires patience and effort.

Life after fasting

Where do we go from here? During the fasting and post-fasting periods you have gained a lot of experience. Take this opportunity to break out of the vicious circle of wrong habits of living and eating.

You will feel that now you have the strength to give your life new directions. Take advantage of it.

- *Take a sheet of paper and write down what you want to change. Do this during the fasting or post-fasting period.*
- *Make a diet plan for the next few weeks and a plan for exercises that suit you best and that you are in a position to do.*
- *In future, try to do without tobacco and alcohol as much as possible.*
- *Help to create self-help groups. Share your experiences and thus help others (see page 69).*

Repeat your week of fasting as soon as your professional or private life allows you to do so. The second or third fast will be much easier than the first. Each fast is different and brings new and interesting experiences. Those who are able to maintain their weight in the meantime, can slim step by step over a number of short fasting periods.

Take advantage of the newly gained knowledge that you can do without food for a period of time while at the same time functioning normally and feeling well.

- *Do not take any meal that you are not hungry for.*
- *Fast if you have a fever, diarrhoea or upset stomach. Your body will reward you.*
- *Plan your next fast now – perhaps together with friends.*

Eat moderately

Continue what you have learned during the post-fasting period: listen to your inner signals. Stop eating when you are no longer hungry. You won't need a Calorie chart, but bathroom scales.

After a fast, a 800 to 1000-Calorie meal will seem like a feast and you will soon have satisfied your hunger. You will feel satisfied and confident that this diet is sufficient, because despite the low Calorie content it contains everything your body needs.

If you do not find this low-Calorie wholefood diet agreeable on a long-term basis, remember the day before the fast. Regularly once a week you should have a day on which you only eat fruit, or rice or fresh, uncooked vegetables. Choose a Monday or a Friday, or both.

Are you among those who get hungry quite often? Then you should eat five or six times a day – small meals chewed well and eaten without hurry.

Changing to a high quality diet

Most diseases that afflict people nowadays are caused by faulty nutrition. We eat great quantities of inferior foods. There is no longer any doubt that pills and injections are not the answer. For all people who are aware of this fact there is only one answer: a change in our dietary habits!

Twelve rules to show the way

Wholemeal bread instead of white bread or rolls. Almost all varieties of whole grains, coarsely or finely ground, can be baked into bread; choose whatever you like best and whatever agrees with you, from rye crispbread to coarse dark bread. Wholemeal breads satisfy your hunger more quickly and for a longer time.

Wholemeal flour preferably freshly ground, instead of white, refined flour. The dark rind of the whole kernel contains high quality oils, vitamins and proteins.

More fresh fruit and vegetables eaten before the meal. Cooking destroys many valuable substances.

Very few sweets and little sugar. Jam, chocolate, cakes and biscuits, all sweetened beverages and ice creams have no nutritional value; if you indulge in them often, they destroy your teeth and your health. Sweeten dishes sparingly with honey, concentrated apple or pear juice, as well as with dates, figs and dried bananas. Diabetics and overweight people should, if necessary, use artificial sweeteners in small quantities.

A minimum of salt, because it retains water in the tissues, favours high blood pressure and therefore burdens the heart and the kidneys. Season with fresh or powdered herbs. Moreover, high quality foods taste good by themselves, so added salt is unnecessary.

Use fats sparingly. Most people eat twice the amount of fat they need. Buy low-fat cheeses and meats, watch for hidden fats in processed foods. Butter loses its quality if it is heated. Use oils and margarine instead of lard or hard fats.

Daily protein intake should be diversified: two-thirds should be obtained from grains and vegetables, one-third from dairy products, eggs, meat and fish. In a vegetarian diet, two-thirds of your proteins should be obtained from vegetables and grains, one-third from dairy products, soya products, yeast and nuts.

Proper combination of food is important. Your daily diet should consist of 12 to 15 per cent protein, 30 to 35 per cent fat and 50 to 60 per cent carbohydrates. Overconsumption of proteins is just as harmful as the overconsumption of fat and carbohydrates.

Choose beverages carefully. What the body really needs is good water. In herbal teas, water is enriched by healing substances and of course, its taste is changed. In soft drinks and fruit juices, Calories are added and so the juices should be diluted by water. Milk is a liquid food and its Calorie and protein content must be taken into account. Coffee and tea should only be taken if you need an uplift, for they are both stimulants. Wine, beer and other alcoholic beverages are intoxicants, depending on the amount in which they are consumed. They are useless for quenching your thirst and loaded with calories besides.

Quality rather than quantity. Do not buy mass-produced meat, fowl or eggs, but try to get free-range chickens and eggs. Organically grown vegetables and fruit not only taste better and are far healthier, they also last longer than artificially fertilized produce that has been treated with insecticides.

As natural as possible. Choose products that have not been chemically treated, for either improved conservation or appearance.

Freshness is all-important. The time between harvest, purchase, preparation and consumption should be as short as possible. This is particularly important for fresh juices and fresh raw vegetables; their taste and nutritional value is reduced in as little as half an hour. Of course, fresh vegetables should always be preferred to canned.

High quality foods every day

Fasting interrupts your dietary habits. After a fast, it is easier to switch to proper nutrition; a change that in the past seemed so difficult. You do not have to change everything at once: do it step by step, but be sure to persevere! It does not matter what your day-to-day life is like. Reflect upon your dietary habits and begin to eat whole, high quality foods every day. You will find some tips how to do it in the preceding pages.

Doing without alcohol and tobacco

Maybe you had been planning for some time to give up smoking and now realize how fasting can help you do it. During fasting everything tastes different. The taste of cigarettes changes as well. Often they will taste like straw: flat, indeed unpleasant.

After not having smoked for one week during fasting, you know you can stick to your resolution. Your non-smoker's training has already started.

During your week of fasting you have proved to yourself that you can live without alcohol. This little break from drinking was not only beneficial for your liver, it also helped your self-esteem. If you are used to drinking alcohol regularly, you are in constant danger of developing a dependency. After not having had a drop for a week, you are now strong enough to take a break from drinking more often.

If your fasting experience has shown that you have a certain dependency on alcohol, do not hesitate to contact Alcoholics Anonymous, a self-help group of people who share the experience and who support one another. Fasting and friends will prove an incentive to seek help. Consult your telephone directory for phone numbers of the groups nearest to you.

Self-help groups

It does not matter whether the problem you have relates to food, drink, smoking or just living – an individual always has to fight harder on his or her own than in a group of people who share the same goal. If you have a problem with overeating you should get together with others who share this problem. In the US and Canada, members of 'Weight-watchers' and 'Overeaters Anonymous' have been successful in helping each other.

Invite other fasters to join you in a group. Tell them about your own experience. Conversation will develop by itself if you have the courage to talk about your personal problems. The others will be encouraged to open up. Don't side-step the issues. You will soon realize that you are not the only one who has problems.

Fasting – a time for reflection

To experience a fast can reach deep into the subconscious of a person, for the experience is also a time for reflection. Besides the physical experience and your attitude about eating, drinking and enjoying various things, there will be a psychological impact which will vary as much as people are different.

Even your first fast will give you an idea that it is possible to find a way to inner freedom and independence of thought and action. The depth of the fasting experience and the scope of its therapeutic possibilities can only be fully realized in a prolonged or repeated fast. If the experience of a week of fasting has encouraged you to try a longer fast, then this book will have served its purpose.

Preventive fasting

Everybody should have the experience of fasting. It is worthwhile knowing that you can live without food for a certain time and that you can learn to eat more modestly afterwards.

I recommend an occasional fast to every healthy person over the age of 30. Fasting weeks for healthy people have proved successful. A group of fasters get together where they live or during a vacation and fast under proper supervision.

After 40, a general 'overhaul' is likely to be necessary, and due to our modern way of life, certainly advisable. Besides fitness training, an 'oil change' in the form of a longer fast is recommended. Prevention is the best form of cure, as we all know. Since prevention is also cheaper than treatment, many health insurance companies in Europe are ready to help finance preventive fasting. Thus they share in teaching their clients how to prevent illness and ultimately the health insurance company gains.

All overweight people should fast. Not only will it help them to correct and control their weight, but they also learn how to deal with their dietary habits and physical disposition to overweight.

All persons who are in danger of becoming ill through diet-related diseases and metabolic disturbances should fast until the risk factors, which can be determined by medical tests, have disappeared, for example in the case of:

- *high blood pressure (hypertension)*
- *elevated blood fats (cholesterol and triglycerides)*
- *elevated blood sugar (beginning of diabetes)*
- *too many blood cells and thickened blood (polycythaemia)*
- *elevated uric acid in the blood (in the early stages of gout)*

In short, anyone who wants to get well should fast. Therapeutic fasting is also recommended as a preventative against cancer, for example, if there has been cancer in your family and you are in a high risk category. Fasting will also prevent premature ageing due to arteriosclerosis.

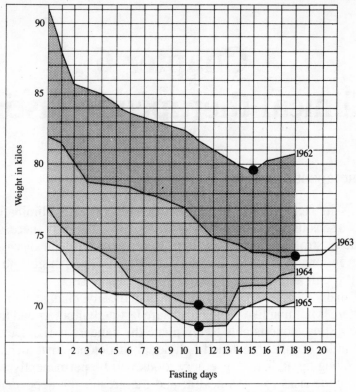

Step by step weight reduction through fasting four times, and moderate eating habits.
Example of a male, 43 years old, 166cm (5 ft 5 inches) tall.
Weight at the beginning of the first fast 91kg (200 pounds/14½ stone) (40 per cent overweight), at the end of the fourth fast 70kg (154 pounds/11 stone) (10 per cent overweight).

- 1962   after 15 fast days, 11kg (24¼ pounds) weight loss.
- 1963   after 18 fast days, 8.5kg (18¾ pounds) weight loss.
- 1964   after 11 fast days, 6.8kg (15 pounds) weight loss.
- 1965   after 11 fast days, 6.2kg (13½ pounds) weight loss.

The above graph demonstrates how lasting the effects of changing one's nutrition and drinking habits can be. In the course of four years and four fasting periods, the overweight problem was reduced from 40 per cent to a mere 10 per cent. In the case demonstrated, it means a total weight loss of over 20 kilos (45 pounds/3 stone), the elimination of the five risk factors listed above, not to mention the overall benefits which cannot be measured by a pair of scales.

Chapter 6
Clinical therapeutic fasting

What is therapeutic fasting?

Prevention is in fact therapy (healing), when it concerns eliminating the early symptoms of a serious illness quickly and successfully. The only successful treatment of heart attacks, strokes, cerebrovascular diseases and vascular diseases of the legs is their prevention. With a lot of patience it would be possible to achieve this prevention through a change in diet and through exercise.

But how many people are truly ready to radically change their comfortable lifestyle? There is nothing like fasting to ensure lasting willpower and inner strength. Therapeutic fasting alone is able to eliminate the dangerous risk factors in a short time and to influence the threatened individual sufficiently that a change in eating habits and giving up addictive or empty foods will be permanently successful.

The greater the risks to one's health, and the greater the dependence on eating habits, the longer the therapeutic fast has to be, along with training in proper eating habits and a healthy lifestyle. A stay of about four weeks in a fasting clinic with specially trained personnel is absolutely necessary.

Therapeutic fasting is more than a fast. It affects the root of the disease and is therefore a causal therapy. What does that mean? Here is an example:

A 43-year-old technician had been a diabetic for the last ten years. His illness caused deep open sores on the soles of both feet; for one year he was unable to work. Despite the best treatment of the sores and a careful monitoring and adjusting of the blood sugar, the sores did not heal. Through a 21-day therapeutic fast combined with a change to a wholesome diet and careful adjustment of the blood sugar levels, the sores healed within four weeks. The man was fully able to return to his job.

Two years later, he was back in the clinic; he had only been well for one year. The reason: weight gain. His lifestyle and his diabetes had got out of hand; the sores on the soles of his feet reappeared. This resulted in one year in a university clinic with careful treatment of the sores, diabetes, diet and the most up-to-date medications. One year of work lost and horrendous hospital bills.

A second therapeutic fast of 21 days with a carefully monitored post-fasting period achieved a weight loss of 14kg (31 pounds/2¼ stone) and a reduction of the high blood fat levels, the elimination of polycythaemia, normalization of the blood sugar levels even though no insulin or other medications were given. The sores healed. Thanks to the new diet and low doses of medication to control the diabetes, the patient was so well that he accepted a job abroad.

With eating in restaurants and boredom in the evenings, he gained weight again. The diabetes was out of control and thus the whole metabolism. There were deposits of fat in the capillaries, especially in the feet. His blood was sluggish, and circulation was therefore affected, and sores that refused to heal were the result. Nine months off the job and more hospital bills.

The third therapeutic fast lasted 25 days, and combined with 15 days for nutritional training was successful as before. Why? Regaining control of the metabolism, thinning of the blood, breaking down the changes in the capillaries. What other therapeutic method could equal this success! The costs were only a fraction of the hospital costs paid the previous year.

Intensive individual and group discussions, diabetic counselling, hands-on training in a teaching kitchen, step by step fitness training – all these measures are employed to help the patient change permanently.

Therapeutic fasting goes to the root of the disease and to the root of one's personal lifestyle. Prolonged fasting of 18, 24, 32 days and longer is *a deep intervention in the metabolism of the patient*. This 'operation without a scalpel' has a great advantage compared to the surgical intervention. Nothing is damaged, yet each cell of each organ, each tiny capillary, each little 'corner' in the connective tissue, where disease causing substances may ever be deposited, is reached. This kind of treatment makes an important difference to people, in the sense that recuperation brings greater self-awareness and an increased feeling of wellbeing.

In the case of allergies and rheumatic diseases, a sustained fast and stimulation of all secretions can change the body's reactions, desensitize it, change the immune system and stimulate the healing process. There are a number of amazing possibilities. One has to realize, however, that they can only happen in a body that is still able to react and not in an organism already hardened by advanced chronic disease.

Therapeutic fasting is thousands of years old. In the hands of an experienced physician and implemented in a clinic it is an amazingly safe, yet effective, therapeutic measure. It follows natural laws of nature. Its value has long been scientifically proven. Anyone who questions this statement simply is not aware of the facts.

Who belongs in a fasting clinic?

The following is merely a list of diseases. Many patients have several or a combination of them at the same time.

Therapeutic fasting is especially indicated in diet-related diseases of the metabolism, and in chronic illnesses.

- *Dangerous obesity – more than 30 per cent overweight.*
- *Diabetes.*
- *Gout.*
- *Polycythaemia (excess of red blood cells).*
- *Fatty liver.*

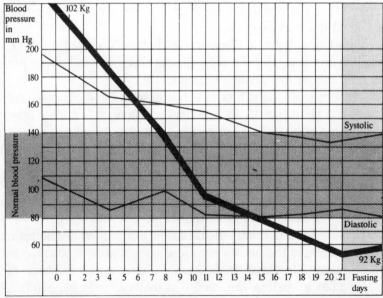

Normalization of the high blood pressure during 3-week fast and associated weight reduction
Source: Dr H. Fahrner

- *Chronic hepatitis (damaged liver cells).*
- *Impaired arterial circulation of, for example, the coronary vessels, the blood vessels of arms, legs and head.*
- *Hypertension.*
- *Risk of cardiac infarction (heart attack).*
- *All diseases where the tissue metabolism is chronically affected, where strong stimulation of the ability to react is necessary, for example in the case of non-articular (muscular) rheumatism syndrome (fibrositis syndrome), rheumatosis, diseases affecting the intervertebral discs and joints (spondylarthritis, osteochondritis, arthrosis).*
- *Chronic skin diseases (eczema, psoriasis).*
- *Venous circulatory problems with open legs.*
- *Allergic diseases of the skin and mucous membranes.*

Many so-called incurable or non-susceptible diseases can be cured or go into remission through fasting and appropriate additional holistic treatment, for example, migraine headaches, chronic headaches, glaucoma in the beginning stages, porphyria, polyarthritis and Bechterew's disease in the beginning stages.

Who must not fast?

- *People without the necessary basic resources: those suffering from malnutrition, people who are physically and mentally exhausted (for example after a long illness or serious surgery). Patients who are losing weight – for example as a result of cancer or tuberculosis.*
- *Mentally ill people, who can not be responsible for their actions. Even so, under the supervision of specialists improvement was noted in schizophrenia and depression.*
- *People who are undergoing great psychological distress, because they lack the inner assurance and calm. In the case of neurosis, psychotherapeutic treatment should accompany the fast.*
- *Those who are physically and mentally overworked should take a week's holiday before embarking on a long-term fast.*

Fasting in a clinic

A certain pattern of fasting therapy has evolved over many years of experience in

German fasting clinics. In such centres fasters live together under medical supervision for periods of three, four or more weeks, and they must accept the house rules which forbid tobacco and alcohol, and which encourage rest in the afternoon and at night. In short, these rules are appropriate to a cure, and the necessary restrictions are offset by cheerful surroundings, bright colours and comfortable furnishings. Fasting clinics should not have a hospital atmosphere.

The fast is followed by a post-fasting diet, with suitable exercises such as hiking, swimming, games, gymnastics in a natural countryside environment. In addition there are facilities for massage, saunas, baths and Kneipp hydrotherapy treatments, along with instruction on correct breathing and body movement. The cultural aspect is also catered for by the provision of a programme of music, conferences and discussion groups – all of which add to the benefits of the fasting experience in German clinics.

The major benefit of fasting in a clinic is the psychological support offered by the experienced staff, and the facilities for diagnostic and metabolic tests to check your progress throughout the programme.

Useful addresses

If you do not know of a physician with fasting experience you may wish to write for advice to:

UK

The British Naturopathic and Osteopathic Association
Fraser House
6 Netherhall Gardens
London NW3 5RR
(Phone: 081-435 8728)

USA

American Holistic Medicine
2002 Lake Street East
Seattle
Washington 98155
(Phone: 206-332-6842)

Canada

Canadian Holistic Medical Association
Box 100-206
2 Bloor Street West
Toronto
Ontario M4W 3E2
(Phone: 416-960-4781)

Australia

Australian Natural Therapeutic Association
31 Victoria Street
Fitzroy
Melbourne

Index